Escape
Points

Escape Points

A Memoir

MICHELE WELDON

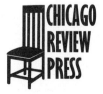

CHICAGO REVIEW PRESS

Copyright © 2015 by Michele Weldon
All rights reserved
First edition
Published by Chicago Review Press Incorporated
814 North Franklin Street
Chicago, Illinois 60610
ISBN 978-1-61373-352-3

Library of Congress Cataloging-in-Publication Data
Are available from the Library of Congress.

Interior layout: Nord Compo

Printed in the United States of America
5 4 3 2 1

For Weldon, Brendan, and Colin, because it is all about you

"*We forget all too soon the things we thought we could never forget. We forget the loves and the betrayals alike, forget what we whispered and what we screamed, forget who we were.*"

—Joan Didion

CONTENTS

part three | **Reversal**

part four | **Overtime**

PREFACE

January 2011

It was a January Saturday in 2011, a home Oak Park–River Forest High School Huskies wrestling tournament with fourteen teams competing in the field house, the squat brick building off the narrow alley where kids tried to sneak in without paying the entry fee at the front door—some parents too, pretending they didn't know about the five-dollar charge when we all know they did. Colin, a seventeen-year-old junior in his second year on the varsity wrestling team, pinned his first opponent in his first match of the day. A wrestler like his two older brothers, Colin was pumped to place, perhaps to win. Confidence was his strong suit.

A local newspaper photographer shot his photo at the millisecond that he pinned his first opponent. I walked over to the reporter to make sure he spelled Colin's name right. The reporters never get anyone's name right; sometimes they get the scores wrong too.

The competition was steep; several wrestlers at Colin's weight were ranked. Colin had earned an honorable mention in Illinois and had just returned from a shoulder injury and three different check-ups with the orthopedic specialist to make sure he could return to competing. The night before he beat the 130-pounder from Downers Grove South at the home dual. I cheered like I was mainlining Red Bull, dressed in orange and blue—the school colors—as my nieces Katie and Maggie shouted Colin's name.

"Go, Colin. Go, Colin, yeah, yeah!" I was videotaping his match from the sidelines, kneeling thirty feet from him.

Now it was noon and Colin was up against a ranked wrestler from Minooka Community High School in the semifinals. Just one minute into the first period, Colin was trying to escape, get his one point—you have to get your escape point—when the other wrestler took him down and slammed him backside on the mat.

The thud was loud, thick and solid like a bag of sand slammed onto the shore. The back of his smooth, blond head took all the impact. And he went instantly limp.

Oh God, oh God.

Colin was not moving.

I dropped my camera and stood. I could see Colin unconscious, completely immobile, out. But in my mind's eye, my mother's eye? I saw him paralyzed. I saw him in a wheelchair, thirty years old. I saw myself pushing him.

These are the visions you have when your child darts into the street, falls off the slide, stands in the high chair. You imagine the worst, the end point, the catastrophe. And you see it—yes, you actually do.

Two matside trainers were trying to resuscitate him with deliberate spiral motions to his sternum. He didn't move. I watched as the coaches surrounded him, all desperately attentive. Colin still did not move, not a muscle, not a hair. All my peripheral vision was erased. I saw only this tight circle with Colin at the center as if it was spotlighted on the stage and the rest of the world went dark. I waited.

He's not moving.

Hail Mary, full of grace, the Lord is with thee.

I held my hand to my mouth so I would not scream. My head and my chest were engulfed in gasoline flames and my hands got hot, damp with perspiration. I just stood there, waiting.

Colin was not moving. One minute. Two minutes. Oh dear God, three minutes.

Parents were mumbling, wrestlers were pointing. It felt as if the entire gym morphed into a hole void of all animation; only the trainers working on him were in slow motion. All I could see was Colin lying on the mat, face up, still not moving, his legs sprawled and his arms at his side, like a Raggedy Andy doll taken down from the cross.

The first part of him to move was his left knee.

I did not rush the mat; I knew Colin would be upset if I did. Coach Mike Powell, the head varsity wrestling coach, who had gone to Colin's side, turned to me and mouthed the words, "He is all right."

"He's moving," a father said behind me.

The coaches helped him up; Colin wobbled toward me. The gym erupted in applause. He looked dazed. Coach Powell walked Colin to the side where I was and I scooped up his sweatpants and headgear, carried his water bottle.

Colin knew his name. He knew where he was. He knew the date.

"Get him to the ER now," the trainer said.

"Someone will get his backpack. Call me," Coach Powell said.

I drove deliberately and calmly to the hospital a few miles away. I was good in crisis. I handled enough of them alone. As a single parent since my boys were six, four, and one, I had been in so many emergency rooms with them so many different times in the last twenty-two years of parenting—stitches, sprains, lacerations, dislocated shoulder, swallowed nickels, yes, swallowed nickels—that I knew how it went. I had good insurance, this hospital emergency room was usually competent and swift, the staff did not make you wait long.

No matter what, it does no good to be emotional, to be upset or distraught or even demanding, you just remain calm. You need the nurses and the doctors to treat you well and your child better. You absolutely do not want to be a pain in the ass. Show your insurance card. Shut up. Do not add drama to the cocktail mix of crisis.

A calm demeanor helped when Brendan nearly severed his left index finger in shop class during his senior year of high school. When the school nurse called me on my cell phone, I was driving down

Sheridan Road to my office at Northwestern University where I was an assistant professor in the journalism school. The nurse was more unnerved than I could afford to be.

"Brendan's hand was severely cut with a blade saw," she said, trembling.

"Is it attached?" I asked.

They must have ice and a cooler and I can be there in one hour, and if they need him to go sooner, for sure, Coach Powell would take him or I could call a friend who might be at home today and I can meet them at the hospital, and it will be fine. You cannot afford to be doused in hysteria; three active sons cure you of that indulgence pretty quickly.

The mother's eye was in full bloom then too; I pictured Brendan with four fingers years down the line, as an adult. I pictured him telling the story to his grandchildren, and then I also pictured it being reattached in surgery. So I have a slew of simultaneous movies playing on screens in my head at the same time.

"He didn't cut off his whole arm, right?"

"Right, it's attached."

I recovered my breath and I knew I just had to keep driving because getting in an accident would be worse. I could call Sue, my nurse friend, and she would call ahead to the ER at Loyola University with the great trauma center I knew well. It was where she worked and everything would be OK; it would just take hours to process it all, get the stitches or whatever else. And then there would be the recovery.

Brendan did not lose his finger. And he later gave me the wooden box he was working on in class; it had dried blood all over the outside. I cleaned it.

Today will be the same. As long as I am not the overbearing mother, everything will go as well as it can. I can stay calm. I only have Colin to worry about today. He is moving, he is talking, he is acting OK. He is not paralyzed. It did not come true. It was the wrong movie.

"Shit," Colin hissed.

He was angry, aggressive, impossible to soothe. He paced in the small curtained-off area where I sat trying to maintain my own equilibrium.

I turned my back to Colin and quietly told the emergency room doctor—who appeared to be at least twenty years younger than me—that Colin was very agitated and not acting like himself. I remembered somewhere from some class, anecdote, website, book, speech, or maybe an episode of *Grey's Anatomy* that a symptom of stroke or something more serious in your brain is a sudden change in personality.

"Do you think you're acting differently?" the doctor asked Colin.

He looked at the doctor, indignant, fuming. "I could have won!"

I sat in the cramped ER space with the blue curtains and scuffed beige walls in complete disbelief. I had imagined his life as a quadriplegic, sipping through straws, and all Colin could think of was not getting a medal at the end of the day.

And he did end up being fine, but it took six to eight weeks, with several visits per week to the concussion specialist at Rush University Medical Center. I tried not to cry when the doctor assessed him by asking him to repeat a series of five or six numbers. And Colin could not.

"Say the months of the year backward starting with October," the doctor said.

Colin could not.

"Repeat these words: *baby, bathtub, ankle.*"

Colin could not.

I didn't cry.

Too much was in the news about concussions: a pro football player committed suicide, the magazine cover story, all of it. I knew enough. All I knew was Colin had to be OK. If I could will him to recovery, I would.

But there was only so much I could do. I could drive him to the appointments. I could wait in the blue fabric chair next to the examining table while the doctor questioned him. I could use my insurance card and write the copayment. I could love him. But I could not heal him from this or from anything. Not today, not yesterday, not tomorrow.

I live in a quiet suburb with wide lawns and thirty-foot trees, a backyard to run around in, a garage filled with bicycles and a basketball net just outside it. I live in a redbrick home with cream shutters and blue striped awnings that belonged to my brother Paul and that my mother helped me buy when I was divorced. I do laundry in the basement, I cook breakfast on the electric stove, and I turn on the thermostat for the air conditioner to kick in during the summer and the heat to begin in winter. In the spring I fill the front porch with clay pots of flowers, which I water daily. I take clippings from the irises, hydrangeas, geraniums, tulips, and coleus in the summer and place them in vases around the house. I lock my doors at night, and the neighbors smile and wave when I pull my car into the driveway. My five brothers and sisters offer me help any time I need it.

That's what you see from the outside.

From the inside, my life would appear as a Rube Goldberg machine with cartoonish and ridiculous gadgets, all moving in complicated trajectories, accomplishing little. That is the easy portrayal, the accepted vision of mothers—and more pointedly—single mothers who work outside the home.

We are seen as holograms of women, eerily transparent visions performing acts of duty in different blocks of time and space, shifting stage sets from work to home and back again. All of it is described with language of desperation and a narrative of drowning—we are made to feel that if we work long hours, we are selfish, and if we spend long hours with our children, we are wasting our brains. And that we never get anything exactly right. It becomes political and polarizing, and it makes you hate the woman next door who drops off her child at school and goes to the gym.

I bristle at the popular cultural notion of single parenting as mine-field, a path dotted with traps, the jeep steered through the maze by the overwhelmed hysteric who needs too much wine with her girl-friends to cope. A woman who can't make it to the meeting or the top of her game, because she has baths to give and books to read to her children. Someone who is always on the verge, always ready to scream because it is all so crazy. There is this idea that a working mother is bound for failure because having it all is a cruel joke, a mesa on the mountain that is unattainable.

I become brittle and defensive when women dig into the barrel of chaotic scenarios to create a story of perennial strife surrounding motherhood, shaking their heads and using *busy* as a four-letter word. It arouses my defenses. You can be busy raising a family; you can also be busy brushing your teeth. Busy is not a bad thing. Sometimes you come home from work after a day that lifts you up out of your shoes and your sons tell you jokes that mentally erase the inconveniences and frustrations from the last two weeks of your life.

We do what we have to do. And the reason it is important to tell the story of someone doing what needs to be done is so the next five hundred women who are faced with challenges see a role model of possibility. That you don't have to be soaked in drama and vodka to cope. That you can maintain your dignity and your sanity, and raise children who contribute to the world while you do the same.

You can do it all. You just cannot do it all well all of the time. And if you really want to give back to your sisters and model for the young women who are most assuredly watching you for clues, if you are seriously considering turning down a promotion or are wondering if ambition is a selfish thing to have, I am here to reassure you that the choice is yours. Trying to make the most of the life you have been granted is a noble thing to do. And the grace arrives.

It does take a village, and it actually takes much more. It takes villagers, family, and someone other than you to show up, really show up, reliably. Sometimes it takes an unlikely stranger.

I knew I could not make up for the father who left my sons. I may never be able to forgive myself for choosing a man who would treat our sons this way. But his story is not mine. Mine is a story of what happens when the door closes and you stand waist-high in the murky puddles brought on from someone else's tsunami. When the shock of the water subsides and you realize you would never drown, you count your blessings.

Because all three of my boys wrestled in youth competitions and high school, I can acknowledge that wrestling has taught my sons a great deal about resilience, integrity, humility, and strength. I am not an athlete, not even close. But the lessons were there for them, and for me as well.

This sport they chose was as much about them as it was about their separateness from me, their single mother, raising them without a father at home, a man whose slow withdrawal from their lives eventually resulted in his complete absence. It was as if after a decade of partial involvement following the divorce, he was gone, like a package lost in the mail without a tracking number.

Wrestling gave them other men to respect, and one man in particular to love. To love like a father.

My sons were wrestlers, and I quickly learned what that meant. A wrestler is a boy who wants to be respected for something only he does. He doesn't want someone to pass, pitch, or kick him a ball. Or a puck. He wants to go out on the mat with no equipment other than headgear and shoes and outwit and dominate with his own strength and agility a boy his size, his age, and his temperament. He wants to be stronger and faster and smarter. And whether he wins or not, he wants to hold up his head, walk off the mat with dignity, and shake the hand of the other coach and the other wrestler. And wait for the next time with a new chance to win.

Yes, it is about dominance, but it is also about owning your every move. It is a sport that offers no shade or hiding place from the singular confrontation before you. Accountability is not optional; your every movement is watched and judged; you are alone on the mat with your training, your strength, your wits, and your focus. Wrestling offered each of my sons something they alone achieved, something they were proud of, something they owned, even if what they owned at times were losses. On the mat, they were young men on their own, showing they could prevail under pressure. It gave them a tribe, made them feel wanted, gave me another way to love them, if only from the sidelines.

In these twenty years as a single parent, I have wanted to prove to myself and to my sons that I could do it all. I wanted to be successful without a partner to back me up. I wanted to show my sons that in spite of setbacks, you can decide that after unexpected losses, life can be predictable. You cannot plan for every inconvenience, major and minor, every betrayal, every loss. But you can plan to prevail.

Millions of women around the globe have steered families to success without a partner. Many contend with dire conditions, unfathomable hardships, and circumstances that are impossible to escape.

Yes, I know I have been lucky.

I have work I find meaningful. I have family that will help me no matter what. I have friends who inspire me and tell me when I am acting stupidly. I have three sons who are exceptional human beings.

Colin healed from his severe concussion. He took the ACT weeks later. He passed his classes. His headaches went away. He applied to the University of Iowa and was accepted.

I heard a story on NPR a while back about a 108-year-old woman who managed to outlive and outwit most of her family and friends. She had what experts called "adaptive competence," a powerful trait that allows and inspires you to view your life as half-full regardless of setbacks. I think I have that. I know my sons do.

Part One

SCRAMBLE

▪ 1 ▪

TRASH

2002–2005

Weldon hurled a new copper-bottomed teakettle into the kitchen trash with a twanging thud.

"Couldn't we just keep it and not think about it as *his?*" I asked.

"It *is* his," he insisted.

It was a Saturday morning in June 2005, and the eldest of my three sons, Weldon, had already spent hours ripping through everything in the house that had once belonged to his father; shoving the old clothes, photos, artwork, letters, blankets, a sleeping bag, and a worn blue comforter into trash bags he took outside and dumped into the garbage cans near the garage.

As a sixteen-year-old high school junior, Weldon did many things that puzzled me. Most of the time I didn't know what bothered him, but he would usually tell me eventually.

It had been a year and a half since my sons' father moved to Europe, eight years since our divorce. Ours was not one of those amicable, let's-stay-friends divorces. It was tumultuous, painful, contentious, expensive. Three weeks after I filed for an order of protec-

3

tion that required my husband to move out of our house in 1995, he filed for divorce and never came back.

To the surprise of everyone who thought they knew the handsome, charming attorney who lived happily with his smiling family in the neat brick Tudor home on the quiet street, my former husband had been physically and emotionally abusive to me over a nine-year marriage. I grew tired of apologies, roses, and promises delivered in counseling offices and at home. There would be no second, third, fourth, tenth chances. I lost the will to try.

I would start over, as a single mother, determined to make a life without fear or uncertainty for myself and my boys, without the unpredictability of a man who could be either the most charismatic person in the room or—to me—the most terrifying.

After full psychiatric evaluations of both of us, and an evaluation by a court-appointed legal guardian, the judge granted me sole custody of our sons, Weldon, Brendan, and Colin, who at the start of divorce proceedings were six, four, and one.

The years following the divorce were not easy but also pretty good considering the complications. I worked hard to stay above water—moving from an adjunct lecturer to lecturer to senior lecturer to assistant professor at Northwestern, contributing columns to newspapers, websites, and magazines; writing books; giving speeches and workshops; and editing other writers' work. I never said no to any offer of freelance employment for pay.

The acrimony between my former husband and me lessened but never disappeared. There was an undulation of empathy, then curt cruelty. I could never predict either. I considered him to be erratic in his attention to our sons; I learned never to count on him for anything related to the boys. He remarried within a few months of our divorce, had a daughter, a half sister to my boys, and in three years was divorced from his second wife.

After that, my ex-husband lived in three Chicago apartments in three years; the boys called the second one the "submarine" because it was a basement apartment with huge pipes across the ceiling. Over the years, I felt as if his presence in the boys' lives was disintegrating incrementally, like a Polaroid photo that extinguishes itself in a closed drawer, the colors fading into greenish-yellow until the image is gone. I could not imagine the long term; it felt obscure, out of reach. His connection appeared to me to be an abandonment, slowly accumulating momentum until, in 2004, he abruptly left the country with a Dutch woman I'll call Ingrid, another one who seemed bedazzled by him. I recognized the signs.

During an otherwise unremarkable weekend visit with the boys in January 2004, their father announced he was moving to Amsterdam in two weeks. The boys were fifteen, thirteen, and ten. I had no hint of his intentions and didn't know what he would be doing, only that Ingrid lived in the Netherlands and had a landscape business. There was some talk about her being involved in seminars on spirituality, but in the months they had been together and the few times I had met her, I admit I paid little attention. Months earlier I had even gone to dinner with her—alone—in an attempt to be cordial. I thought it might make the visits with the boys and their father go well if she was there.

Apparently, the day their father announced he was leaving the country, he loaded his pale gray Chevy van with trash bags filled with most everything the boys had ever given him—the Father's Day presents from kindergarten, their homemade paintings, cards and photos of themselves. He told the boys to keep it all for him *in case he came back*.

Then he dropped them off at home with all his leftover reminders of their childhoods thrown into plastic bags. I was not home to catch them in this latest freefall; I had gone to dinner with a friend. That Sunday night I walked in the door and saw piles of boxes and trash bags stacked in the front hall. The house was quiet. The boys were in their rooms.

"Whose stuff is this?" I asked when I reached the second floor. Knowing they would never go on a cleaning binge without several months of daily prodding, I was confused.

"Dad's," Colin said.

According to Colin, their father had said that the reason he was moving to Amsterdam was because all he did every other weekend was watch their wrestling tournaments, football, basketball, and baseball games, and help with homework. His life was much bigger than that, he told the boys.

Mine is bigger because of that, I thought.

I walked downstairs, my heart pounding, furious. I called my former husband on his cell. "What did you do?" I shrieked.

He told me he was building a better life for himself. He was no longer a practicing litigating attorney, having left the large firm in Chicago years earlier. He became a salesman for energy products, then a salesman for something else, I never really knew. I only knew he paid less in child support every year, until he paid nothing at all.

Whatever he did offer was never enough to cover the child care for the boys while I worked—the string of a dozen women over eighteen years to be my backup before and after school, 6:30–8:30 in the mornings, and 3:00–6:00 in the evenings. They would walk out the front door when I walked in the back door; sometimes they made dinner. Sometimes they made the beds. Sometimes they took laundry soap in plastic bags for their own laundry, and sometimes they forgot to pick up a child at practice. Sometimes they made chicken noodle soup that made the whole house smell like heaven.

My former husband had sold the blue striped couch I lent him for his apartment, the one that my mother had given us when we moved back to Chicago. He kept the $200.

This move to Amsterdam was all for our sons, he told me on the phone, though he offered no specifics about how that would work or how it would include their school and sports, their friends, or any part of their lives. It was like I was listening to a random caller to a radio talk show spouting off claims that I knew were improbable. He said he was giving them the opportunity of a life in Europe.

"They have a life here," I said.

How in the world would I pay for them to have a jaunt in Europe? I was able once to eke out a trip to Disney World with the boys, but that was because I signed up for a junket where I had to sit through hours of sales pitches for Disney time-shares that I had no intention or wherewithal to purchase. A European adventure was not a priority. Getting them through high school and college was higher on my list.

Even though Weldon's first year of college was more than two years away, I had an instinct my ex-husband would not honor college payments from our divorce decree. I just knew it, the way I know how a movie—especially a Lifetime movie—will end a half hour into it. That is why I worked for a university—for the portable tuition payments, among other things. I had worked at Northwestern for ten years before Weldon went to college. I qualified and my boys would reap the benefits: 40 percent of tuition paid to any university for twelve years of college for the three of them.

"You needed to let me know, to prepare them. This is a lot for them to take in so suddenly," I said.

How would I make up for this? How would I spin it so the boys wouldn't feel their father was leaving them? All their gifts in trash bags. Once again, it was up to me to absorb the aftershocks.

I never could have foreseen his choice. Not from the man who was effusive and gregarious when we'd married in 1986. Not the man my friends said was a real catch. I know that it sounds absurd, but how he behaved, who he appeared to be, his abuse—it surprised me.

Four months after our wedding, he struck me for the first time, on the chest. We went to a marriage counselor, and I believed my husband when he said that all he needed to do was calm down before he came home from work. For the next nine years I believed what he said to the three therapists in three cities we lived in—Dallas, South Bend, and Chicago. The first move was for my career; I was recruited to be a feature writer and columnist at the *Dallas Times Herald*. The second move was for his decision to go to law school; the final move was coming home to raise our children near our families. I bolstered my faith in the in-betweens—the times between the episodes of physical abuse—when he professed devotion and sincerity, the times we worked to create a family. But the in-betweens were as consequential as vapor, as amorphous and illogical as an ill-conceived wish. That was a lifetime ago.

The summer after his father left for Europe, I agreed to let Weldon visit him there for three weeks. I was careful to be supportive; I helped Weldon pack, gave him a credit card for emergencies, and bought him a leather photo album for all his photos of the trip after he returned. I would not obstruct a relationship with his father.

Two weeks into the trip, Weldon called from Florence, Italy.

"Where is the David?" he asked.

"The Michelangelo statue?"

"Yes." His voice sounded odd.

"It's in a museum." I couldn't offer more concrete help just then; I'd last seen the iconic statue of a young, naked David, arm poised to sling a rock against Goliath, when I was twenty-three and on a three-week Italian tour with my friend Mariann.

"We are trying to find it. Can you tell me how to get there?" Weldon asked.

"It's been more than twenty-five years; I can't remember. It's on a side street in a small museum, but everyone will know. Just ask, or look it up online." I couldn't look it up for him right then because I was away from my laptop. I didn't know whether to laugh or worry even more. Of course, I worried more.

We chatted a little and he said he was fine. But the call was so strange; his voice was hesitant. I had given him a credit card in his name on my account—so I could track where he was. Of course, my ex-husband offered no itinerary. I didn't know where they were going, when, or for how long. Weldon was only fifteen. But I could call my credit card company and check on recent charges he had made and where. Luckily, he used the card almost every day—for food and incidentals. If I didn't see a charge, I worried. There were several days without charges when I was extremely anxious and imagined the worst.

"If something happens to Weldon, you will hear," my sister Madeleine assured me.

As far as I knew, not finding the David was as difficult as it got.

Weldon returned home on the prearranged flight days later. Brendan, Colin, and I picked him up at the international terminal at O'Hare. We held welcome signs and a balloon. Weldon brought home gifts for each of us—a small bud vase from Delft, Netherlands, for me, T-shirts for his brothers.

It took Weldon three years to tell me how strange and hurtful the trip had been for him. He said his mission had been to convince his father to come home—if not for him, then for Colin, who was ten years old at the time. It took him even longer to tell me that his father had left him for two days in Italy with a stranger because he needed to go back to Ingrid.

Weldon told me much later that the trip made him feel he was capable of solving problems and managing on his own—that if he could be fifteen and left alone in Europe by his father, he would always be fine. This is not a lesson you want your children to have to learn.

"Why did you get rid of everything that was your dad's?" I asked Weldon after the clearing out episode. "And why now?"

"I don't want anything that was his," he said. "When I asked him why he ignored Brendan's graduation, Dad said, 'What does that have to do with me?'"

For Brendan's Roosevelt Middle School graduation a few weeks earlier, the boys and I went to dinner in Old Town to celebrate. When we got home, there was no phone message waiting, no e-mail, no congratulations card in the mail from Brendan's father. His aunts and uncles on his father's side sent checks. I bought Brendan a new suit, plus a battery-powered stuffed dog wearing a mortar board and a sash that said GRADUATE. The dog danced to the verse, "The future's so bright, I have to wear shades" when you pressed the button on his chest.

In 2002, the boys' father was still living in town and seeing them mostly every other weekend. I was visiting my mother in her small room at Kindred Hospital, just a few miles west of our house down North Avenue. The boys were at home with a sitter I had paid to spend the night, the same one who stayed the night when I traveled for work about once a month.

My five brothers and sisters and their spouses, and the hospice nurse, were at the hospital too. We had been there all night. We didn't want to watch our mother die. But we stayed.

As we sat or stood near her bed, next to which were small resin statues of Mary and Joseph on the nightstand, my mother took a loud, labored, rattling breath; opened her eyes wide; and looked off to the left. A huge smile engulfed her face, as if she was seeing something or someone. She closed her eyes. We waited for her next breath, but it never arrived. The nurse came in the room; they were monitoring Mom from the nurse's station.

"Your mother has passed."

We all stayed in the room for a while, said the Rosary together one more time, and cried. I looked over at my mother lying in her bed, her arms quickly turning an odd slightly bluish tint, until a nurse covered her with a sheet.

After another hour, my brothers and sisters hugged and kissed each other good-bye and we all left the hospital. I walked to the parking lot with my sisters Maureen and Madeleine and Madeleine's husband, Mike, feeling that helplessness I felt when my father died in 1988, as if I'd been dropped from the roof of a building without a net below.

"Are we orphans?" Maureen asked.

"I don't think adults can be orphans," Madeleine answered. "Only children can be orphans."

The boys were already at their schools; the sitter who had spent the night got them ready, packed their lunches, and drove them. I went home and called my ex-husband from the phone in the breakfast room where I had painted on the wall the Chinese proverb, "Govern a family as you would cook a small fish—very gently."

"The boys will need to go to the wake tomorrow and the funeral the next day," I said. "They can't go to Wednesday night dinner with you; they have to be at the funeral home."

I felt like I was on autopilot; I hadn't slept. I guess I hoped that he'd respond with compassion and kindness. My mom had just died, a woman he'd known his whole life who had been friends with his parents since they went to college together. So I let my guard down, pictured myself speaking to a friend, to the man I wished he was. I said something stupid, something I didn't really mean. I was tired. I was scared.

"When I am ninety-five, I am going to spare the boys what I just witnessed and step in front of a moving train so they don't have to watch me die."

He laughed. "Don't worry, Michele, I will shoot you long before then."

2

SUNDAYS

2000–2008

The father bent down at the edge of the mat and screamed to his son, "Crush his face! Crush his face!"

Brendan, who was eleven, looked up at me, his left arm twisted like a wet kitchen towel by this bloodthirsty boy who appeared to be a mini-assassin.

"Excuse me, this is his first match ever," I said. "Does he have to crush his face?"

The father glared at me as if I was speaking in tongues.

At every Sunday youth wrestling tournament, hundreds of boy bodies in shapes from gangly to marshmallow were bare-armed and categorized from forty pounds to more than two hundred, ages five to fifteen. There could be as many as one thousand youth wrestlers at one tournament and at least twice that many parents, grandparents, and siblings. On Sundays the gyms in every city and every state around the country were tropically humid and alive with an unforgiving drumming of shouts, grunts, and whistles. It sounded as loud as if I were sitting in the last row of a 747.

Two years earlier in 2000, as a sixth grader exhausted by the daddy-is-the-coach syndrome so dominant in the suburb where we lived, Weldon read a brochure mailed to the house about folkstyle youth wrestling offered at the local public high school. He did not want to play on one more team where the coach's son got the key positions and the most play time. Sure, some moms were coaches, but I could not take the time from work, and I never could have been able to coach a sport for all three sons, which was the only fair way to do it.

"It doesn't matter who your father is in wrestling," a friend told me when I explained how Weldon had picked this sport new to our family. "It's just you on the mat."

So I signed him up that October for the Little Huskies Wrestling team at Oak Park and River Forest High School and sent in the check; he began four evening practices a week that sometimes ran until 9 PM. After practice, Weldon would come to the car exhausted and wet with sweat, but smiling. I had to bring Brendan and Colin with me in the car to get Weldon; they were ten and seven years old, and I couldn't leave either home alone. Sometimes the three of us tried to predict exactly what time Weldon would emerge from the field house or the precise outside temperature registered on the dashboard of my Volvo station wagon.

"Two degrees!" Colin would say. Some nights he was right.

When Weldon folded into the front seat, his duffel bag behind him, I asked how it went.

"It was hard, but it was great."

That first year of youth wrestling for Weldon, I felt like Jane Goodall observing wild chimps: an awkward outsider, not knowing the scoring, moves, what to cheer and when. I was ignorant of the unspoken mother's law that you never, ever approached a son who had just lost. You waited for him to come to you. And then you just listened. I wondered why I had never known about this vast secret underworld of competition for the very young, a different universe from other sports. Like swimming, track, or gymnastics, you stayed all day for a tournament. But unlike any of those, that day consisted of sometimes brutal one-on-one contests against someone aimed at slamming your son to the ground and pressing both his shoulders flush to the rubber mat.

I learned the mythology around competitive youth and high school wrestling was steeped in error. There was the common misunderstanding that it bore a resemblance to the idiotic, clownish, steroid-soaked freak fights of platinum blonde professional WWE wrestling on television. There was also a homophobic taboo about young men who loved the sport, including mockery and taunts from kids in sports with less close contact—say tennis or lacrosse. I was learning more each week.

Yes, there were wrestling moms filling the seats in the stands, yelling their sons' names, but most everywhere you looked—on the gym floor, in the cafeteria, in the stands—were fathers and sons. Fathers embracing their sons after a win, fathers putting their arms on the shoulders of boys after a loss.

In the early years after our divorce, my ex-husband would take the boys to wrestling tournaments if they fell on his visitation weekends. But he was never there consistently. Not every time. Not every match.

Looking around the gyms, sometimes the sons resemble their fathers so much—the slope of the jaw, the shape of the arms—that it is startling. Just observing the legacies makes me feel a lot of things, not the least of which is my somehow being responsible for what my boys did not get, that I made the choice to marry someone who would go away. That I married someone who would willfully hijack my sons' feeling that they are loved unconditionally by both parents. I could do my part, but I could never do both parts.

The first portion of the morning consisted of weigh-ins when hundreds of boys, and a few girls, were weighed in a separate gym from parents, accompanied by coaches, then grouped by age and weight, their weights drawn on their arms in marker. I noticed on one boy about eight or nine years old, the number 172 was drawn an inch or so high in wide, black permanent marker strokes on his upper right bicep. The way his pale flesh folded and blossomed from beneath his shiny polyester singlet made him look as if his body was filled with scoops of cookie dough. Behind him was a father with the same furtive expression and rumpling build, his thick hand firmly gripping his son's shoulder.

The wrestlers were grouped by weight and age so the first two-minute period with thirty seconds of rest followed by two one-minute periods—with thirty seconds of rest in between—were evenly matched. Unlike high school and college, youth wrestlers didn't need to make a specific weight; each wrestled what he weighed that morning and was grouped with other wrestlers in that weight and age bracket, say a weight range of 106–108 pounds.

Some of the compact boys in the "midget" category had muscles so sharply formed and legs with distinctly circular calves that they looked like animated resin trophies, caricatures of miniature men. I wondered if they considered the political incorrectness of the midget category and if they would eventually shift to call the category "little people."

Boys darted through crowds standing in line at the refreshment stand or on the gymnasium sidelines, holding green or blue liter bottles of Gatorade, their hair buzzed short and purposeful, waiting for volunteers to sell them hot dogs, pizza, pretzels, donuts, popcorn, chips, or bagels with cream cheese. Their fathers were either elated or furious, some wearing XXL T-shirts stretched taut like drum covers over their bowling ball bellies. Mothers wore T-shirts with photo likenesses of their wrestlers.

In that bewitching morning hour before the wrestling began, mayhem reigned on the mats with dozens of wrestlers running in circles, jumping on each other, having chicken fights, stretching, doing jumping jacks, running in place, playing tag—all of them all at once. "Eye of the Tiger" was usually playing over the loudspeakers; it was the unofficial wrestler's theme song. If you could've harnessed the raw energy in the gym, you could've saved the planet.

Parents chatty and amicable in the early morning settled into their stakeout sections, club teams seated with their wrestlers in the stands, stepping over McDonald's bags and Dunkin' Donuts boxes.

The most coveted spots were in the top row against the gym wall for back support. Those wall slots filled up quickly on two sides of the gym. Some of us brought the inexpensive portable stadium seats we bought at Home Depot. If you were lucky, you might be able to find an electrical outlet for your laptop. Chances were there was no Wi-Fi. I brought dozens of papers to grade for my freshman journalism class and, in December, stacks of Christmas cards to address. I brought to-do lists, newspapers, and magazines to read. I created current events quizzes.

"Save me a spot," I said to Caryn, who had three wrestling sons of her own, two out of her three boys the same ages as my boys. Our youngest sons, Colin and Sam, would later be inseparable best friends.

Usually, the matches were in a Chicago suburb perhaps thirty miles away and far outside my comfort zone; finding the high school only with the help of Yahoo! directions. Without a GPS, using only printed instructions, I often had to retrace my steps after mistaking a right for a left, trying desperately to remember where I spotted the last Starbucks in which strip mall near which bank. Sometimes I thought MapQuest and Yahoo! made intentional errors in the end of a trip—a left instead of a right, a north instead of a south, Glenbard East High School instead of Glenbard North—just to force drivers to pull into a gas station or 7-Eleven to get help from a clerk, who was hopefully over sixteen and knew the names of the major roads. I once asked a young clerk where the local high school was, and he replied that he didn't have any idea. I asked someone in the parking lot on my way back to my car, and she motioned that it was a block away.

"What are you doing Sunday? Can you meet for an hour for coffee or something?" my sister Madeleine would ask.

"No; I'm watching wrestling."

The eight or so youth tournaments each season were on Sundays because high school gyms were used for team varsity wrestling and basketball on Saturdays. Like Weldon before him, Brendan was part of Little Huskies, an offshoot of the Oak Park and River Forest High School team and one of the organized clubs that served as feeder pipelines for high school wrestling programs across the state and the country. Every week about a dozen to twenty young boys from our team wrestled, many of them the tail end of wrestling families with older brothers in the sport.

Few champions started the sport their freshman year of high school; many had been wrestling since grade school, some since kindergarten in these Sunday youth wrestling tournaments. Plenty of these boys attended supplemental private wrestling training programs twice a week all year; at some the cost of one-on-one training was one hundred dollars an hour. For groups of two to three young wrestlers, it could cost sixty dollars an hour per wrestler. I could never afford to send the boys to these elite team programs—I had neither the time nor the money to get them there. But plenty of parents did; and their kids usually won the tournaments, the state titles, the scholarships to Big Ten colleges.

As the day matured, the air grew dense and humid with the feral odor of pizza, hot dogs, and sweet, ripening sweat, the intensity thickening and festering by midafternoon. Families arrived with Igloo coolers of food like Cheetos, pork rinds, and peanut-butter-and-jelly sandwiches; separate bags of knitting and crossword puzzle books; and smaller children in car seats and strollers. Some parents left intermittently to smoke in the parking lot.

No matter how much food was brought in, it seemed so much more was purchased and so much else thrown away. Sometimes a few high-protein, low-calorie offerings were available from a concession stand, like oranges and bananas, but most of the food was deep-fried and cheesed. There were mountains of candy choices. Long, colored sugar ropes hung from many boys' mouths to their waists as they gobbled their way to the end, like a long wick of a cartoon bomb fuse.

At some concession stands you could find the walking taco—an opened bag of Fritos with a scoop of hot chili poured on top and a teaspoon of shredded cheddar cheese, with a plastic spoon plunged into the chunky mess. I made hundreds of them working the food line at Little Huskies tournaments. You needed a Crock-Pot to heat the chili and ice to cool the bags of shredded cheese. And lots of paper towels.

The announcer gave the predictable procedural details and then played a recording of "The Star-Spangled Banner," sometimes the recording by Whitney Houston, most of the time just a recorded instrumental version with a church organ. Refs blew whistles, and the wrestling matches erupted on four rubber mats with each mat divided into two. Two wrestlers were on each mat. Red and green strips of Velcro were fastened onto the boys' ankles just before their match—the same Velcro strips used over and over again on different wrestlers—to differentiate the wrestlers for scoring. I used to wonder what the bacterial count on those strips would be at the end of the day—and then I wouldn't let myself think about it. The ref wore one red and one green wristband and held the corresponding colored wrist in the air to quickly note the points scored for each wrestler.

In the matches, the boys looked like dancing spider monkeys on fast-forward, rolling over each other, grappling, shooting for a takedown, pinning, standing up, crying, winning, arms shot in the air. The thuds of an official pin—a referee's slam of his open hand onto the mat signaling a boy was pinned and the match was over—occasionally pierced the air like an exclamation point. The smallest and youngest wrestlers were first. Some were so cute they looked like Power Rangers dolls, some cried inconsolably when they lost, and others were cocky and determined, like small pit bulls. The matches worked up from the youngest Midget through Novice to the Cadets, some of whom at fifteen had been wrestling ten years and looked mature enough to father children. Some even sported facial hair and tattoos.

"Now you won't take first," a father reprimanded his son, as if he had just committed a felony. The boy's shoulders were shaking from crying, his neck and arms red from the recent loss. The wrestler made his way to a corner of the gym to cry.

Each mat had a nearby long, folding table where up to four score-keepers sat, controlling the clock and the score. One mat was connected to the overhead scoreboard; the other matches were scored on foot-high cardboard cards of numbers that scorekeepers—usually high school volunteers—flipped forward on double rings to show points earned. Every match had its own digital running clock. Occasionally a parent shouted at the ref to contest a point.

"Parents off the mats, only wrestlers and coaches on the floor," the announcer pleaded often each hour. But it was as futile as trying to stop passing drivers from watching the twisted remains of a car crash.

In the stands, boys slept like young cougars between matches, curling onto pillows, hooded sweatshirts pulled over their heads, covered by down-filled coats brought hastily from home, water bottles strewn like spent rifle casings across the floor near the orange peels and candy wrappers. A young wrestler could have as many as six matches in one day, fewer if he lost early on, more if he won. The goal was not to go home early. The goal was to go home later sporting a green ribbon with gold-colored medal for first, second, or third place.

I always waved at Weldon. I called his name. Mostly he ignored me. He had mastered the expressionless chin chuck, lifting his chin in acknowledgment in a quick upward jerk. Brendan did it too, then Colin.

But as a parent, you didn't go for the acknowledgment; you couldn't. It would be too upsetting; the immediate return on investment could not be measured. You went because there was no other activity you needed to do to catch up on work, run the house, or God forbid do for yourself, that was more important than being there in that gym for that child that day. Unless you had two other gyms to be in for your other children; then you did your best to catch a piece of everyone's glory. You went because you believed—had to believe—that years from now when you were gone or when they were much older, they would remember the sight of you in the stands in the team colors screaming their names. And to them it would be a good memory.

You want to contribute to the good memories.

Your children will never recall happy memories of you getting a manicure or staying home to read a book. I felt I had a finite window on the timeline, minutes between the beginning and ending buzzers,

to show them I cared enough to be there. I could get myself a manicure and read a book when they were all away at college.

With prodding from the announcer, the wrestlers in the appropriate age groups headed to the holding pen with their coaches, and
officials called their names for check-in at the assigned mat number.
They attempted to put novice against novice and veteran against
veteran. It was no fun to beat someone easily. You wanted your
matches to be tough. Team parents kept track of who on the team
was wrestling when and on what mat.

"Is Brendan up next?" Caryn asked, and then we would all move
together, sometimes with Leslie, Paula, and a few other moms to
get closer to the mat where he was wrestling and cheer for the few
minutes or less it took to declare a victory or a loss. And we would
all do the same for each other's sons. Some high schools wouldn't
ever allow you on the gym floor, and if so, we watched from the
spectator's gallery above; hoping not to stand next to the parent of
the child our son was wrestling. If one of the team moms was not at
the gym for the tournament, another mom would give her a play-
by-play by cell phone: "He's looking real strong, they're circling,
the other boy shot, got him down, he got out, one escape point,
they're circling . . ."

Each of them called me about Weldon, Brendan, or Colin if I
was in traffic or couldn't attend because of another commitment with
another son somewhere else.

More than a few of the mothers on other teams were dressed in
spandex-tight jeans and low-cut camisoles as if they were headed to
a night on the casino boats, while some wore baggy sweatshirts with
the youth team logo, their long brown hair sprayed into ponytails,
bangs sitting stiffly on foreheads. One woman we nicknamed "Hot
Mom" because at these tournaments she gave her son back massages
between matches, so exaggerated and sensual it made us squirm.

One father wore a T-shirt that read, IT'S NOT THE SIZE OF THE
DOG IN THE FIGHT, IT'S THE SIZE OF THE FIGHT IN THE DOG. The
Little Huskies logo is that breed of dog, standing upright on two legs
and looking menacing, more human than canine. Most of the logos

for other youth teams were bulldogs, raptors, wildcats, or wolves. Some used a skull and crossbones for their logo. The teams had names like Force, Predators, Wolverines, Rhinos, Gladiators, Iron Men, and Grapplers.

CHAMPIONS ARE MADE, NOT BORN, read another T-shirt. A young boy carried a plastic bin of round yellow nacho chips smothered in bright orange melted cheese to his place in the stands. WILL TRADE SISTER FOR HEADGEAR was his T-shirt pronouncement. I'D RATHER THROW YOU THAN KNOW YOU, one team's shirt read. Colin said he was sure they didn't mean it but wore it because it rhymed. Another young man's shirt said something about how basketball players play with balls, but wrestlers have them. He walked by too quickly for me to see it all.

"Stand up! Get up, get up!" a mother screeched to her son locked helplessly in a cradle hold on another mat.

"Drive! Drive! Drive!" a dad in warm-up pants and a baseball cap shrieked to another wrestler on a different mat. Dozens of video cameras were aimed at different contests.

"Two!" one ref shouted with the whistle clenched between his teeth, two fingers raised in the air for the scorekeepers when one wrestler had a takedown—when a wrestler successfully gets the other wrestler down and prone on the mat. When the match was over because of a pin or the clock ran out, the wrestlers removed the red or green Velcro straps from their ankles and placed them on the center of the mat. Whistles blowing, it began again and again. Parents screamed, "Pin him!" or "Stand up!" what sounded like thousands of times during the day.

A wrestler in an emerald green singlet who looked about twelve or thirteen years old landed on his wrist in a fall. His arm snapped midway up his forearm, bending it at a right angle like a chicken wing. We all gasped in the stands when we quickly learned what happened from whispers moving through the crowd like a wave. The match stopped; the young wrestler lay on his back silently until the paramedics arrived and placed him on a stretcher after immobilizing the right arm. He was stoic, not crying but wincing. Throughout the gym, parents stood and applauded as he was rolled outside. Dozens of wrestlers in primary-colored singlets watched nervously. The wrestling continued.

When Colin was wrestling as an eighth grader at 103 pounds, a boy about his age with short dreadlocks sat near us sporting a black baseball hat with fourteen orange safety pins tacked on the side.

"What do the pins mean?" I asked.

He looked astonished. "It's for every pin I have this season."

Weldon told me repeatedly that I asked dumb wrestling questions.

To me, it seemed as if in every match my sons were proving they were different types of men altogether than the father who left them.

"That's silly," Weldon told me later. "You can't think about anything like that, you can't be distracted, you have to focus or you lose."

For Brendan, wrestling transformed him from an ill-at-ease middle schooler tenuous in sports and necessarily suspicious of the social spiderwebs, to a comedian in peak physical shape who dared to prove to himself his own strength. He did imitations of most everyone on the team and the coaches.

For Colin, his first sport of choice had always been football, but during his freshman year, wrestling eclipsed that passion. Colin wrestled only part of two youth seasons in seventh and eighth grades. He won his first match in a pin—I have the photo—and lost the next few. He was not an immediate fan of the sport.

"I had some sweaty guy's crotch in my face," Colin reported to Weldon after his first youth wrestling match.

"If you're any good, that doesn't happen to you," Weldon said and walked out of the room.

My sons were wrestlers, and to them and their friends I was a wrestling mom. I was not a university assistant professor, an author, a journalist, a sister, a friend. I was in their world every weekend and I was a spectator; I believed in my bones that my presence mattered. Even if all I got was a chin chuck at the end of the day. I needed my sons to know I was paying attention; that I wouldn't leave, that nothing was more important to me than they were.

I expected to spend my weekends watching wrestling most of the year. We drove to the suburbs forty miles away and sometimes flew to the regionals and nationals one thousand miles away. We stayed at the Clarion Hotel or Ramada Inn if it was an away tournament and drank the bad coffee in the lobby, where they served bagels if you were lucky and donuts if you weren't.

When I met another woman anywhere—on a business trip, in line at the movies, at a conference or a party—who mentioned her sons wrestled, we both knew what it meant. We understood the pre–weight-making mood swings, the nervousness before each match, the sweetness or sullenness after, how they looked like gladiators when they competed and tired puppies on the long ride home.

"You're a loser! You're a loser!" one mother from another team seated about three yards from me in the stands screamed at her son as he slowly approached her. He was sweating and breathing heavy, fresh from a loss on the mat. He looked to be about seven.

"What is wrong with you? Don't even talk to me, don't even talk to me!" she insisted. "You should have won!"

My stomach tightened. Not one of the women sitting near her from her team blinked. The boy placed his headgear down beside her and walked away, shoulders slumped and head lowered.

Sometimes the greatest lessons you learn are what not to do and who not to be.

■ 3 ■

PROTEIN

1990–2010

As a toddler Weldon placed on the pediatrician's growth chart in the seventy-fifth percentile for height, twenty-fifth percentile for weight.

"Put some cream cheese in his scrambled eggs," the doctor suggested. "He needs more fat in his diet."

For the next eighteen years he grew taller while staying lean, a perfect genetic makeup for a weight-making wrestler. When he hit preschool I stopped making him scrambled eggs every day and he grew into the practice of craving an enviably balanced diet of meat, vegetables, fruit, potatoes, pasta, and bread—lots and lots of whole wheat bread. He didn't ask for candy, french fries, and all the other childhood junk staples. When his friends were driving their parents crazy with a low-tolerance appetite and a narrow menu of macaroni and cheese and hot dogs, Weldon wanted grilled vegetables. And sushi.

"Fun Lunch" was launched every Friday at school when Weldon and Brendan were in fourth and second grades. Every week a rotating fast-food menu of burgers, chicken nuggets, or pizza was brought in by a group of hearty mom volunteers. You had to pay extra for it, of course.

"I don't think they should eat fast food so often," I wrote to the principal. "It can't be good for them."

As the lone conscientious objector in the entire school of kindergarten through fifth grade, I lost the argument and succumbed to Fridays of junk. According to the boys, being the only student in the cafeteria with a homemade lunch on Fun Lunch day would be one step up from being homeschooled. The only thing worse would be if I was a Fun Lunch mom volunteer, they said, or if I was like any of the other moms who volunteered in the office or the library every day.

"Some of those moms need full-time jobs," Colin said in first grade. The mother of one of his classmates hand-delivered her son a thermos of hot soup every day at 11:15 AM. Colin was mortified. I considered him evolved.

It seemed that even as a preschooler, Weldon—more than my other two boys—was hyperaware of meal ingredients and preparation methods. If food was deep-fried, baked, or overprocessed, he didn't want it. He asked me, the waiter, hosts, or whoever set food before him what was in the food and how it was prepared. Years before he began wrestling, Weldon had a phenomenally mature "my body is my temple" approach to what he ate. His diatribes on my daily diet soda and morning coffee seemed a little over the top. He clucked his tongue when I bought spinach dip. You would think it was atomic.

"You know that isn't good for you, right?" he would ask. And he was seven.

At ten, he presented me with a three-page typewritten argument for purchasing a water filter for the kitchen, citing the health benefits. He e-mailed me dietary suggestions—I should eat more blueberries, more salmon. Not those turkey or soy sausages for breakfast. One birthday he bought me vitamins, three enormous bottles of them. Flaxseed oil was one. That was better than the birthday present Colin and Brendan bought me the same year: conditioner for "extremely dry, damaged hair."

"Isn't that the kind of hair you have?" Colin asked.

For what I thought was convenience for me and a helpful fund-raiser for the school, I began ordering frozen food through Market Day—a nationwide movement to give schools a percentage of sales on frozen convenience foods ordered by school parents.

You may have seen the trucks with the red apple logo or the signs on school lawns that read MARKET DAY PICKUP TODAY. Weldon objected to every monthly Market Day offering I ever ordered, from the chicken Kiev to the ravioli and breakfast burritos. Appalled, he would read the multisyllabic ingredients out loud and gasp at the sodium content. You would think I was offering him cyanide.

"If you're so picky, you make dinner," I told Weldon.

And he did on occasion. Weldon's red bell pepper soup was better than any I had ever enjoyed in a restaurant. He started with chicken broth and added pureed and sautéed red peppers and yellow onions, carefully following a recipe he found online. His carrot cake was moist and delectable, even though he somehow got grated carrots on the ceiling—every time.

The other boys helped too. I figured this was a good by-product of having a working mother. Train a generation of men to cook.

Brendan took up grilling; his favorite thing to do was marinate— fish, chicken, or beef, it didn't matter. He would have a dozen bottles of spices, oils, and vinegars set before him on the cutting board island in the kitchen and mix them all up. He, too, would neglect to put anything away. Or wash the pans.

Colin joined in as chef; his specialties were scrambled eggs; pan-cakes; hot sandwiches with melted cheese; tuna salad with cilantro; spinach sautéed with olive oil, garlic, and lemon; and grilled aspara-gus with balsamic vinegar.

Between the diet of gross reality shows they all devoured (the ones with a circus of dysfunctional families or the skateboarders who wrecked houses), all the boys watched cooking shows. Brendan had a crush on Rachael Ray. Weldon bought me cookbooks and read them himself.

"We totally smashed that," Colin said. That meant they ate it quickly, not that they squished it on the walls, which is what I feared at first.

Food appeared to be more important to them than most anything else. Outside of wrestling season, I could not stock the refrigerator or freezer fast enough. Three gallons or more of milk a week, four boxes of cereal, two loaves of bread, pounds upon pounds of chicken, turkey breasts, ground turkey, steak, lean ground sirloin, pork tenderloins, salmon, pasta, oranges, bananas, spinach, broccoli, tangerines—the boys could eat a wooden crate of about thirty tangerines in a weekend. Four pieces of fruit a day per boy.

I worked primarily to pay the food bill. And the sitter. And the mortgage. Yes, I worked for my own professional highs, but the paycheck was spoken for before it arrived.

I would stuff the refrigerator on Saturday morning when I came home from the grocery store, and on the following Thursday night the naked shelves held only olives, pickles, mustard, barbeque sauce, and vitamins plus low-fat hazelnut-flavored coffee creamer. After dinner, while we were all doing the dishes, Weldon and Brendan would stop to stand before the opened refrigerator door and graze.

"We just finished eating," I said. "You can't possibly be hungry."

But they were. If it wasn't processed, canned, or frozen, or if I made it from scratch, they would devour it almost without chewing. Each one of them would ask for seconds, rave about how it tasted, thank me for making it. They loved it all—the roasted chicken; the turkey meatballs; the homemade apple pie I made with butter, cinnamon, and apple cognac; plus the fudge brownies with a dash of lemon extract.

"They're good eaters," my mother had remarked about the boys. They ate first, asked questions later, and tried anything.

This constant, daily stream of affirmation was a very good thing; I cooked, they ate, everyone was happy. I was a good mother making sure my boys were healthy. They smiled at dinner. Each one of the boys would eat as if he was on fast-forward, often finishing the entire meal before I even sat down.

"Wait for MOM!!" Weldon would shout at the other two—after, of course, he had downed several bites.

I clearly stated my objection to two-handed eating, one hand gripping a fork and another hand with a knife at the ready. Like Popeye.

"One hand," was my abbreviated reminder.

I reprimanded them over what I called shoveling—introducing new bites of food before the old bites were chewed and swallowed.

"You're shoveling," I would say, trying to model appropriate dinner etiquette. "Put down the fork and chew. Wait. Wait. Wait."

Then I threw in what I considered the clincher. "Women would prefer to eat across from someone who was not acting as if he was in a hot dog–eating contest."

Sometimes I thought they were afraid there would never be another meal after this one, and that if they did not eat the last chicken breast, sparerib, or baked potato, another brother would get it and they would lose out. Only the alpha male won the food. If I made chicken pot pie for dinner, or turkey chili with three beans, the first son up the next morning would finish it off before his brothers could slip the bowl of leftovers into the microwave.

"I have thirteen muffins in my cargo shorts," Brendan announced in the van.

We were in Florida visiting my brother Paul one spring break and were headed back to his house after dinner at a salad-and-soup buffet restaurant. When we got to Paul's, Brendan emptied his pockets and put the muffins in a bowl on the kitchen counter. They were all gone by the morning.

I wondered what all this consumption really meant; if there was some deep psychological need to nurture themselves with food, if they were overcompensating for something. But they didn't horde food, they didn't eat in secret; they just ate a lot. They worked out three or more hours every day. Sometimes I swore they each consumed up to five thousand calories a day.

There is a primal relationship between a mother and her children's nutritional intake. Without exaggeration, my sons' lives depended on the food I provided.

When each boy was an infant, I worried at first about where I would breast-feed him every hour and forty-five minutes. Then when they were toddlers, I packed enough formula and crackers, Ritz Bits, or Teddy Grahams in plastic sandwich bags in the diaper bag to get through a few hours. Then I graduated to making sure they each had a good lunch packed for school—sandwich, fruit, pretzels—which I made the night before to avoid the morning chaos.

I aimed to give them a balanced dinner when they came home each night. Working every day, the healthy sit-down dinner was a challenge. A few of the sitters would cook dinner—chicken soup, broiled vegetables, and whatever meat I defrosted in the morning. But most of the sitters over the years refused to cook. I prepared enormous amounts of food on the weekends—meatloaf, turkey burgers, chicken breasts—to last through the week. My sister Madeleine invited us for dinner most Sundays and gave me the leftovers. If family parties were at Maureen or Paul's house, they sent me home with enough ham, bread, cheese, and coleslaw for a few meals. It was understood my sons ate a lot.

I offered my boys soup, crackers, and Jell-O when they were sick, and cake on their birthdays. I limited fast food, pizza, and the boxed mac and cheese with the bright yellow-orange powder. I did my best to make sure what I put in them was good for them. It's what I called a mother's high; I literally watched them bloom. They grew taller, they stayed healthy; it was simple cause and effect. Good diet plus multivitamins and you were on your way to the good mothers' hall of fame. Well, that was the hope.

Every other part of parenting seemed less straightforward, more fraught with emotion. But this? Feed them good food and they are happy? That seemed a no-brainer.

So it was unsettling as a mother of wrestlers who loved to eat to continually witness the finite wedge of time—before and after matches, season after season, from November to March (longer if they wrestled off-season)—when they deliberately and pointedly restricted their intake and disciplined themselves ounce-for-ounce to make weight, to be the exact number of pounds in a weight class in which they would be certified to wrestle. It was a loaded issue for me as a mother who had basically been on a diet for thirty-five years. Give or take twenty pounds, I have been the same size since my late twenties—I won't say since college, because I was about twenty-five pounds lighter at that time than I am now. I didn't know whether I was impressed or terrified to hear a son say he dropped five pounds during a three-hour practice, when it would take me forty days and nights on a treadmill, eating only ice chips, to do the same thing.

When I lived through the sixteen or so weeks of limited consumption that constituted Weldon, Brendan, or Colin making weight, I admired them for their intense discipline, especially when I could not walk past a bowl of onion dip made from the soup mix without sampling. But it also was frightening; I did not have control over what they did. I had to let them go, I could not care for them in this basic way and none of them would listen to me about it anyway. They were going to make weight no matter what I said or did. And I could not stop them. It was for wrestling, it was what they needed to do.

A vegetarian, Coach Powell told the wrestlers how to identify what food was good for their bodies. Work out more, be smart, run a mile or two, he told them. He gave them printouts of diets and a booklet on healthy eating.

"Skip the cheeseburgers," he said.

I told the boys my brother Paul's simple rule: don't eat anything you can't wash. That would eliminate desserts and include pretty much just meat, vegetables, and fruit. I tried to do the same.

Though he started wrestling in high school at 119 pounds, Weldon wrestled at 140 pounds in his junior and senior years, a weight he maintained in season through daily workouts (weight lifting and running), eating protein bars, and having the discipline it took to excuse himself from eating most everything at Thanksgiving meals—no dressing, no mashed potatoes, no gravy, just PowerBars and lean turkey. That's right, not even pumpkin pie.

During season Weldon said he was never completely full; he would go to sleep hungry, wake up hungry, and stay just a little hungry for weeks on end. At five feet ten, his weight was less than what I weighed at five feet six. Whenever I said I was worried about him or suggested he could at least eat something—a small piece of chicken, a banana, something other than a Clif Bar—he was irritated and reminded me yet again that I didn't understand because I was not a wrestler.

Brendan started high school at 165 pounds at five feet four, got down to 135 his sophomore year at about five feet seven, then voluntarily catapulted into the practice of gaining thirty or more pounds after season and losing that much before the next season. The summer before he was a senior, Brendan was up to 195 at close to six feet. By November he wrestled at 171, where he stayed throughout that summer.

Colin weighed 123 at the beginning of his freshman year, having started in youth wrestling at 80 pounds. He wrestled his freshman year at 119 and sometimes bumped up to 125 depending on what holes the team had at what weight. A few times he wrestled at 112. Almost immediately after his sophomore varsity season, Colin weighed 140 pounds. His junior year on varsity, he wrestled at 130, sometimes 135. Before wrestling season began, he weighed 142. At times he would drop up to eight pounds in one week.

This severe yo-yoing was not something I could do quickly or chronically. I spent several months in Weight Watchers a few years ago and lost seventeen pounds. I have kept most of it off, but with enormous effort. My boys could lose seventeen pounds in a week to ten days. Every season. During wrestling season weight was a daily conversation centerpiece in our house, as was the protein and caloric measure of every morsel of food. It was an odd contrast from the abundance of food they required the rest of the year. After season, they could each eat a pint of Ben & Jerry's with a spoon while standing.

"Don't eat that, man," Brendan would say to Colin.

"What? A grapefruit doesn't weigh much."

"The water in it is heavy. Have a grape. Tuna."

And on and on the arguments went. Over almonds and ice cream and pasta, the virtues of protein shakes and the evils of chips.

The boys each said they could tell how much anyone weighed by looking at him or her. Feeling unusually confident, I asked the boys once how much they thought I weighed. They were excruciatingly right, but I did not let them know that; some numbers a mother prefers to keep from her sons.

For years I believed my sons went through all of this as a vainglorious attempt to prove something to other people, to show them they each earned their victories without nepotism or favoritism. But I have come to believe they did it all for nobody else; not for me, not for the coaches or the crowds in the stands. I believe they did it not to exorcise anger or frustration or to prove their worth as athletes. I believe it was to prove to themselves that they could maintain self-control and perform alone without anyone else's intervention—on a treadmill, in the weight room, on the mat against one opponent, or at the dinner table facing a steaming Thanksgiving buffet.

As their mother, watching weight-cutting was like watching each one climb into a wooden barrel and throw himself off the edge of Niagara Falls. It was counterintuitive; I was here to provide them sustenance. As their mother I wanted them to be full—of life, of food, of love, of dreams, of laughing memories. So it was hard for me to step back and let them do this. But I did. I understood deadlines and I tried to apply that personal sensibility to their weight-cutting. They had to meet the weight requirements on deadline, just as I had met my word requirements on deadlines for almost thirty years.

A long time ago I held each son in my arms as a newborn and nursed him; it felt so daringly, secretly complete. The process was universally enormous and personally miniscule at the same time. It was me, just me, in this perfect symbiotic exchange with each one of them, and each of us was fully sated. What I had for them was what they wanted and needed. It made me feel real power, not power I had over them, but power I had from them. No one else could give them that, and no one but my sons could give that to me.

Every few weeks, then months, I would take each son to the pediatrician for a checkup and he would be measured on the same kind of scale they use to weigh tomatoes or eggplants at the farmer's market. And he would always be bigger. Gained two pounds. Gained three pounds. The nurse would remark on how great that was and he must be nursing well, congratulations. It was good for him, it was good for his immune system, keep going.

Thankfully, that equation got intensely more complicated with each passing moment of their lives. The world began to fill them up; it was no longer that simple equation of two. I would never step back in time to that era, not even for a millisecond, nor do I miss it. But it was disorienting years later knowing that each son got on the scale every day before and after practice, trying to get smaller and weigh less, and working that hard to make a certain wrestling weight. But it is what they did. They did it for themselves, for the team, yes. It was about asserting self-control. Yet, a side effect of all the training and making weight was earning the respect of Coach Powell. They did not want to disappoint him.

▪ 4 ▪

COACH

2003–2009

I called Coach Mike Powell and asked him to help. I had the high school head wrestling coach on speed dial, as did most parents of wrestlers on the team, all of the wrestlers, and many of the wrestling alums. By 2007, he had been Weldon's coach for the last three of four years, and Brendan's for the last year. A few nights earlier Brendan had pulled a stupid teenage stunt and I was at the end of my mother rope. It had been eleven years since my divorce, and about that long since I was able to ask for any paternal backup. Besides, their father had been living in Europe for three years by then.

"I'll drive over in about an hour to talk to him," Powell offered. "Have Colin there too. He should hear this."

When Powell—that's what we called him around our house, just one word like Cher, Madonna, Elvis, or Usher—arrived at our house that June night in 2007, straight from a workout, he asked for a glass of water.

"Don't hug me, I'm sweaty," he said when I answered the door.

Weldon and I sat on the couch with Colin. Powell was perched on the edge of the red Chinese Chippendale chair; Brendan sat across from him in a matching chair. Although he was in his early thirties, Powell looked at least ten years younger—baby-faced with dark eyes underneath wire-rimmed glasses, sporting a dark mustache and goatee. On his head were outbursts of jet-black hair; it had grown out since he shaved his head bald with the team just before Thanksgiving—an annual team ritual that made for rotten family holiday photos. The wrestling season haircut is why we posed for holiday pictures in the summer.

Powell talked for close to an hour, his voice deep and low, forceful but not punitive, looking directly at Brendan. And Brendan looked straight at him and stayed silent, nodding, listening, not lowering his eyes or walking away, the way he did when I confronted him. With Powell it was eye-to-eye.

"It doesn't matter in the end what kind of wrestler you are," he told Brendan. "It matters what kind of man you are." He paused. "I love you no matter if you win or not. But the point is to be a good man."

And then he left.

"Good to see you in practice," Powell wrote on a brochure for wrestling camp he sent to Colin as an eighth grader when he worked out with the team off-season.

Colin broke his collarbone on the first night of that summer's wrestling camp; a much heavier boy slammed into him against the wall during a game of tag before wrestling even started. Powell called to tell me to get to the high school right away and take him to the emergency room. Later that night, Powell called to check on him.

"Let me talk to him," he said. "I feel so bad."

In a photo in his bedroom, Weldon is wearing his blue-and-orange singlet, still donning the blue plastic headgear, just having leapt off the mat into Powell's arms after winning a key match at state in February 2007. He is shining with sweat and Powell is cradling him.

The grin on his coach's face is best described as gritty, solid joy. This one photo reminded me of all I ever wanted for my children, a moment when I knew they were loved fully. Look, see, he is loved.

Powell was almost godlike to my boys, and not just to mine; almost every parent on the team had what we called Powell stories. He drove immediately to the home of one boy who was a victim of a violent crime; Powell talked to him for four or five hours.

"Powell was the only one able to calm him down," his mother said.

When Peter Kowalczuk, the heavyweight cocaptain of the team with Weldon, made it to the Olympic Trials in Las Vegas in 2008, Powell was there coaching him and cheering him on. Sometimes I thought I must be idealizing who Powell was and how much the boys depended on him. And then Powell did something Powellish—like have the wrestlers sandbag the local Des Plaines River all day because of threatened flooding.

Powell called if a wrestler missed weight lifting to see what was wrong. If nothing was wrong, he chastised him but was never demeaning. If Powell heard rumors of a boy drinking or getting in trouble, he called him into his office and told him he had to stop or he would be off the team. The boy would stop.

"You can't lie to Powell; he knows when you're lying," Charlie Johnson, another wrestler, told me. The four other wrestlers in my family room one Wednesday night nodded.

There was no deterrent for any of them stronger than the disfavor of Coach Powell. A mother or father could threaten taking away driving privileges or a cell phone, even grounding indefinitely, but nothing mattered more than the possibility that Powell had lost respect for the boy. In five years, no wrestler had been reprimanded at the school for a violation of the code of conduct. You couldn't say that about members of the other sports teams.

Whatever Powell said held a hundred times the weight of a parent, teacher, anyone. The boys craved his approval. They would do anything they could for him. I was sure it was one reason he was named Coach of the Year in 2009, a statewide honor for all high school coaches.

"About damn time," he said half-kidding.

It was the start of the 2008–2009 season, and I was waiting for Colin to emerge from the field house at about 8:30 PM after practice. I congratulated Powell on his award as he headed to his car, the end of a normal fourteen-hour day for him.

"Colin looked real strong tonight, real good," he said. And when Colin got in the car a few minutes later, I told him.

"Powell said that? He did?" Colin smiled ear to ear.

In the daily practices the boys said they worked harder than they ever thought possible, with a half hour of jogging around the wrestling room followed by more specific wrestling drills, followed by almost an hour of live wrestling—intense matches between wrestlers of similar weights. Two and a half hours of practice without breaks every day, each wrestler dripping with sweat; Powell and the coaches too. My sons would come home with their practice shorts and T-shirts in tied, plastic grocery bags. When I opened the bags to throw the clothes in the washing machine, they would be soaked through as if they had been dropped into a lake. A few times Brendan left his workout clothes in the trunk of the car in the winter, where they froze as solid as bricks.

Sometimes Powell would tell the boys practice was going to be short that day, and when he pushed the boys harder, he smiled and said, "I lied." Later he told Brendan, "If you want to be a badass on the mat, decide you are a badass. That's the difference."

About five feet ten, Powell weighed about 180 pounds, not much heavier than his high school and college days. He was in peak shape, muscular and cut, able to wrestle with the boys and able to beat all of them any day. At the wrestle-offs for the varsity spots before the 2008 season, an exhibition parents attended, Powell wrestled Ben Brooks at the 189-pound spot. It was close, and Ben won.

I congratulated Ben immediately after. He looked up and smiled, "He gave it to me. He let me win."

It was Powell leading the other coaches to push the pace, wrestling with some of the upper weights himself, demanding they keep trying for takedowns, keep sticking it out. At least one wrestler broke down in every practice, crying or fighting with another wrestler, but Powell told him to keep wrestling. And he would talk to them in his own code, "You dig?" he would ask; or "Legit," meaning one of them did something that won his approval.

"You go through hell in that room," one wrestler said. "He makes you want to do it. I work that hard, we all do, just so he could say to you, 'Nice job.'" He added, "You keep sticking it out because you know you're going to be a badass. No one on any other team has a warmup even close to us. They're all gassed. It makes you feel so good about yourself."

The first two and a half hours of practice were the workouts; the last hour and a half was Powell talking to them about life. They called them "Powell lessons," and he told them about mistakes he made, how "he screwed up," all in a way that the young men could hear. "He would give you a rib shot and then give you a dead serious talk," one wrestler said. "He tries to be our friend and coach and mentor at the same time," another said.

I remarked to one of Brendan's teachers at the parent-teacher conference in his senior year how much Brendan liked and respected Powell.

"All those boys think Powell walks on water," she said, rolling her eyes.

"I am not so sure he doesn't," I said.

Before every match began, he embraced Ellis Coleman, a nationally ranked wrestler who eventually became an internationally ranked wrestler aiming for the US Olympic team, and kissed him on the top of his head. Ellis eventually made it to the Olympics—London 2012. Powell was there. Both Weldon and Colin were there in London to watch Ellis as well.

Powell drove Ellis's older brother, Lillashawn, to college his freshman year and moved him into the dorm. He advised all the young men on the team on everything from strength training to nutrition to girlfriends.

"No fake sugar." He said it so often, the wrestlers wanted T-shirts made with the slogan.

One summer night in 2008 Powell drove to Peoria—about 170 miles each way—to pick up Ellis and Lillashawn, both wrestling in an off-season tournament, after their grandfather had died suddenly. Their mother couldn't make the trip to retrieve them.

Powell contacted all the team members and caravanned with the boys to the wake a few days later. When another wrestler's father died from a long-endured brain tumor, Powell was there, rallying the boy's teammates to his father's wake and later funeral. Two boys who quit the team in their junior year came back to the team a year later.

"I'm sorry, Coach," Powell said Jake Venerable told him on the phone.

"What weight will you wrestle this year?" another coach asked Ellis about his varsity plans for his senior year.

"Whatever Coach Powell tells me," was his answer.

In weekly e-mails to the team's families, Powell saluted the boys by name for specific victories or struggles and signed each e-mail, "In relentless pursuit." One e-mail read, "The coaches could not be more proud of our guys. The athletes have really dedicated themselves; working hard, sacrificing, displaying courage daily. What a great group of young men."

"I was always defined as a wrestler," Powell said. His nickname as a kid was Mikey Powerful.

As a kid, Powell said he was high-energy and tried karate as a way to deflect some of that nervous velocity, and also Boy Scouts, but neither outlet worked. His father, Bud, started him in youth wrestling when Powell was a forty-five-pound first grader; the next biggest wrestler was almost twice his weight and in fourth grade. Powell stood his ground. His parents divorced when he was a teenager, and he says it was wrestling that got him through it.

I was hoping wrestling would do the same for my sons.

After winning the Illinois high school Class AA state championship at 171 pounds in 1994 as a senior at Oak Park, Powell went on to be an All-American at Indiana University. Following graduate school, he began coaching and teaching at his alma mater. His father volunteered alongside him for every tournament, victory, and major team event.

He hosted team members to live with him and his fiancée (later his wife), Elizabeth, if the wrestlers were having a tough time at home and needed help with homework or staying out of trouble. Even after he was married, he spent as much time as ever on the team; he had barbecues for the boys in his backyard and arranged for fundraisers like the June car wash or a community trash cleanup to get them better equipment or fund a trip. He set up tutors for team members if they were doing poorly in school.

"My job doesn't have boundaries," Powell said. "With these kids, the more you invest emotionally, the more you see is there," he said.

On New Year's Eve each year, he made sure one wrestling family hosted a party for all the wrestlers so no one could get in trouble and attend a party with alcohol or drugs—which would result in a dismissal from the team. Weldon's teammates started a Facebook group their senior year, WWMPD, standing for What Would Mike Powell Do. During season he brought the team to Bikram Yoga classes on Sundays. He taught them how to breathe deeply to relax. He talked about the environment.

"Next year we'll be sure to have environment-friendly ink on the team shirts," he said.

Powell followed up and followed through, more than you would think possible for a coach who met these teenagers for the first time when they walked into his wrestling room the first day of practice. He talked to them like a friend, not a youth minister. He spoke their language, cursed sometimes, didn't hold back, didn't preach. On the Huskies wrestling website was the tagline, "In Powell we trust." He was almost too good to be true.

"He invests his everything in us," one wrestler told me.

Powell brought the team from not being ranked in the state to being team state champions, undefeated for the season in 2009. The team was awarded a trophy with all the wrestlers' names engraved on the front. It was the first team championship for the school in more than a dozen years for any sport, and the first ever for wrestling. They came in second in 2012 as a team. In 2014, the high school team was ranked first in the state. In January 2015, the team was ranked number one in the country.

Before the team drove to the individual state championships in 2009 at the University of Illinois, the boys got their money together to buy Powell cigars to celebrate the victories they knew would be theirs. They collected enough money from each wrestler to buy a cigar for everyone on the twenty-one-man roster plus the coaches. Brendan drove to buy the cigars, bringing with him his glass change jar filled with pennies, nickels, and quarters. They were still little boys, now doing big man things.

"Call Powell and tell him," I said when Weldon told me the news that he won a prestigious scholarship to study abroad the summer after his college freshman year.

"I called him first," he said.

Weldon even walked like Powell; the wrestler's walk, spine straight, shoulders pressed deliberately back, head held high, arms poised just slightly away from his sides as if he is wearing an invisible holster—*High Noon* meets the Olympics. He walked with motion generated from the hips, not bowlegged exactly but with his legs pushed outward from the knees and his upper body held still—*Riverdance* on Muscle Milk. A lean, taut confidence.

You could spot the young wrestlers by this walk anywhere in any city. They were marked by thick, strong necks and backs, not as much bulk as it was a muscular control of the space they occupied, Hummers in a parking lot of Nissans. It was mass minus body fat, size without excess. It was a different walk than a swimmer's or a football player's; the carriage showed more pride than bravado, with a gymnast's ease and a weight lifter's strength.

The walk was not robotic but intentional and aimed, although we did nickname one of the wrestlers from another school RoboWrestler because he looked as if his limbs were made of metal. Each of his steps seemed studied and precise, as if he was walking on the mat for the first period of the first match, when anything was possible and the red digital numbers on the scoreboard read *2:00.* Three two-minute periods, six minutes of intensity. They all wrestled hard, whistle to whistle. Buzzer to buzzer. It wasn't over until then. You keep wrestling. You stand up. And if you get taken down, you stand up again.

During a match, Powell would shout so loud at the wrestler on the mat, telling him what moves to do next—to takedown, shoot, pull his head up, get his arm out—that he was always hoarse at the end of the dual or the tournament. Powell was often voiceless after meets, after hours of jumping up from his seat at matside and yelling instructions. The wrestlers looked up if they could and watched what Powell motioned for them to do. At the end of a match, even if the wrestler won, Powell was there to demonstrate what he could have done better. If the wrestler lost, Powell was there to tell him what to do next time.

"I can only hear Powell's voice when I'm wrestling," Weldon told me once.

"When I am on my deathbed, I will be the proudest man because I gave everything to everything," Brendan said he told the boys at practice.

Each summer Powell and three other coaches took the wrestling seniors, from the 103-pounder to the 285-pound heavyweight, on a weeklong backpacking trip, a teambuilding exercise planned and executed with the help of assistant coaches. Weldon and eight teammates went to Glacier National Park, where they climbed blue-white mountains and talked about everything in life beyond wrestling. Brendan and his teammates went to Zion National Park in Utah, where Brendan said they ate peanut butter quesadillas atop red mesas and talked about what it is to be a man who earns respect.

Weeks in advance, Powell sent home detailed lists of what the wrestlers needed to bring for the trip—backpack, sleeping pad, Nalgene bottles, sunscreen, flashlight, cash. Knowing teenage boys the way he did, he had them all bring their packed gear to a meeting three days before departure to double check. These life-lasting memories of landscapes off the mat were the backdrop for the boys' later imitations of Powell sprinting up the side of a mountain with all his gear plus tents, first aid, and food—perhaps one hundred pounds of equipment in all.

My three boys had dozens of coaches in other sports throughout the years, but the boys were not nearly this close to any of them. We certainly never quoted any of them at dinner.

When my sons were younger it was all I could do to get them to their practices with the help of sitters during the week, and in the evenings and on weekends sit and watch the games, matches, meets, and tournaments. I made a master list of the boys' baseball games and practices one season when all three were playing house league baseball—forty-eight practices and games in all. Some at the same time. All on three different fields. During the week, the sitters helped. Some Saturdays, games were spread out from 8 AM to 3 PM. Some Saturdays, all three games were at 9 AM, so I drove from one field to the other hoping to catch at least an inning where that son did something he wanted me to see.

Weldon never really clicked with any of the coaches on the local baseball, basketball, or traveling soccer teams in grade school or middle school. They yelled too much, were dismissive, or didn't seem to care personally about him. And the truth is they probably didn't. They had their own kids, their own work, their own lives. You couldn't expect anything beyond the game or the tournament. And a few said as much. They were speed fathers, like speed dates, who could provide for hours a week what an absent father could not. And nothing more.

Brendan liked a few of his baseball and basketball coaches and only one of his soccer coaches. He played his last year of baseball in sixth grade when his coach called him a derogatory name at practice. He played youth football from third to eighth grade, and one year he liked his football coach a lot, talked about him often, but when the season ended, the relationship ended.

Colin had devoted coaches for many league and traveling teams from baseball to soccer to basketball. For two years Colin had Tim Odell as a youth football coach, whom he adored. Colin told me once he decided he wanted Tim to be his father, partly because of how kind he was to Colin and partly because he had his own Super Bowl ring. I said we would need to ask his wife.

I never threatened the boys with a coach's name the way I did when I said, "Stop, or I'll call Powell."

Powell arranged parent night every first Monday of the month in season at a local pub. Whoever could, showed up. We ordered sandwiches, burgers, beer, and salads and talked. It was a way for families to come together, a tradition Powell initiated. We had new T-shirts each year that read, HUSKIES WRESTLING FAMILY. It was a way for all of us to take responsibility for each other's sons.

"Our goal is to be a place where kids feel special, empowered, and loved," Powell said. At the wrestling banquet during Brendan's senior year and Colin's freshman year, Powell talked about each wrestler on the team from freshmen to sophomores, junior varsity and varsity, with personal details and often some jokes.

He teased one wrestler. "Ninety-five percent of the time this kid drove me nuts," Powell said. "But he worked hard and would do whatever the team needed." Powell embraced him.

He told each wrestler how proud he was of him. Parents fought back tears.

"We believe 100 percent in what we do, this year the kids believed in what we do, and when you all believe in that, it's a powerful thing," Powell said.

The back table in the south cafeteria was laden with homemade dishes—the families of juniors and seniors brought the entrées, the parents of the freshmen brought appetizers and salads, the parents of sophomores, desserts. After the wrestlers and their parents heaped lasagna, fried chicken, casseroles, and vegetables onto paper plates, and plucked brownies and cookies from trays and platters onto separate plates, Powell spoke from the podium's microphone.

"This is the hardest sport for a parent," Powell said.

The parents nodded. It was hard to get up at 6 AM to drive them to weight lifting, make lunches before the tournaments, endure their weight-making moods, get them to the team bus every Saturday morning, and sit in the stands and watch for up to six hours at a

time—fourteen hours if it was a regional, state, or national tournament. And when your son got to the mat, you might be watching
him lose or get hurt. There was more work than glory, especially
since you traded hours and hours of support for just a few minutes
of watching him in competition.

Powell continued his talk from the podium. "The coaches work
the hardest, but we get the most out of it. We call it a wrestling family because in a lot of ways it is a family. By no means do we intend
to replace you as parents, but it's nice to be loved."

He added, "Thank you for giving your sons to us."

5

EAR

December 2004

Weldon stood in front of the bathroom mirror one morning exclaiming, in what I identified as a tone of glee, "I'm getting it! I'm getting the ear!"

I was mortified. I inspected it and promised I would look it up online and see how to proceed as soon as I got to work. His ear was puffy, enlarged, swollen with blood. It was gross. Midseason of his junior year on varsity and his fourth year of wrestling, he was getting it. I called Powell, sure that this would excuse my son from practice and upcoming matches for some time if not forever. He's getting the ear, for goodness sake. The ear.

"It's not a big deal," he said.

I knew what the ear meant. His coaches all had the ear. Usually, the pair, like Powell. Misshapen and noticeably nonsymmetrical, no two cauliflower ears manifested the same way. Some were outright horrific, elfin, pointed, and enlarged—years after the trauma. Forever.

Were athletes who played volleyball so permanently changed? Swimmers? Some ears were just rounded and reddened, like mini water balloons. Others more grotesque, with the unpredictable crannies and bumps reminiscent of the plastic-molded models of mountains and volcanoes used in elementary school geography class.

It was called cauliflower ear. But cauliflower was bland, pale, unremarkable. The name implied none of the mother terror it inspired, and none of the mysterious pride wrestlers associated with, well, this deformity. It scared me. And I wanted to do everything I could to prevent it.

Would people stare? Would they consider him defective? Was it my fault?

"You'll want your girlfriend or your wife to like your ears," I said to Weldon when I could think of nothing else to convince him it was not a good thing.

"I won't be with a woman that shallow," Weldon responded.

It was an acquired condition that came from repeated trauma to the ear, resulting in hematomas and a collection of blood and fluid that permanently damaged its structure. It was something wrestlers got after having their heads pulverized against a wrestling mat over and over during the course of several years, creating severe friction and a breakdown of cartilage. And for reasons I could not understand, wrestlers didn't apologize for it, hide it, or shrink from it. They wanted to get it.

It is what they got when they did not wear the headgear in practice that was required in folkstyle competition. They did not wear it off-season in freestyle or Greco. To me it would be like lifting a pan out of the oven without wearing oven mitts, knowing your hands would burn and blister and it would hurt, but you did it anyway because you believed it meant you were a good cook. Season after season they skipped the headgear no matter how many times their mothers made them swear they didn't. Cauliflower ear was not for the accidental wrestler, it was for the wrestler who saw the sport as something far more than six minutes of competition in a singlet. It was for the real wrestler, the one who believed all those sayings on the T-shirts, like GO HARD OR GO HOME, PAIN IS WEAKNESS LEAVING THE BODY, or TAP OUT OR PASS OUT.

The affliction was painful and impossible to disguise. If the athlete wore his hair below his ears to cover it off-season, then maybe you wouldn't notice. But in season, long hair was not allowed, or at least not encouraged. If a wrestler had long hair, he was required to wear a hair cap. It would seem common sense to attempt to avoid getting cauliflower ear. But like so many aspects of all three of my sons' lives, this acceptance of the injury was anathema to me. Like the calluses on the hands of an expert shoemaker, cauliflower ear showed the world that you wrestled with everything you had, and a little thing like a permanently deformed ear would not dissuade you from the sport. Wrestling mattered; the cosmetic appeal of your ear didn't.

Weldon's teammate, Peter Lovaas, a 145-pounder his senior year, earned himself the ear. He said he told women he met in college either that he was attacked by squirrels, or that he rubbed peanut butter on his ear for his cat to lick off. Sometimes the cat nipped, he said. All of the girls recoiled.

Wrestler ear, boxing ear, or rugby ear were emblematic of all I found counterintuitive and all that I knew instinctively about trying to keep my boys from harm. Weldon earned the ear in his junior year. Brendan earned the ear the next year, his sophomore year. Weldon's right ear and Brendan's left, with shifting lumps and swollen tissue, were visible reminders of all that was startlingly different about us: their maleness and impulsivity, their determination, lack of vanity, and a burning dedication to a goal regardless of price.

The ear meant I failed. Their disfigurement was all my fault; both those ears were my fault.

To a wrestler the ear was a sign not that you were less than perfect, but that you were committed to the sport. It was about manhood and drive, an outward sign that you were someone who suffered for greatness. This was the exacted cost, and it was small compared to the monumental high of having a striped-shirted referee thrust your hand in the air in victory over your most fierce opponent. It was a sign. You were good and you wrestled for a very long time. Or you had soft ears susceptible to this injury, Weldon told me. Some people just have soft ears.

The second day of his engorged ear, I took Weldon to the emergency care center near our house. It was the spot I called the drive-through doctor or Doc in the Box—where I took the boys before or after work in emergencies and upon suspicions of bronchitis or infections. It was open from 7 AM to 11 PM and was able to do X-rays and stitches, a much better option than my pediatrician's office, which was open only from 10 AM to 4 PM, timing that was after I left for work and long before I got home.

"This is stupid," he said on the ride to the immediate care site.

Weldon was clearly annoyed and I was surely a pathetic, overprotective mother for making him go to the doctor in the first place. Heck, he could just stab himself with a needle and puncture it, drain it, and be done. Weldon continued with his usual you-wouldn't-understand-you-are-not-an-athlete diatribe. His coach told me all it needed was a draining. Weldon at first said the trainer would drain it in the wrestling room that afternoon, and I cringed. He came home from school with it undrained. Then he asked me to please just get a needle and drain the blood from his engorged right ear. I almost puked. As if I would take a needle and poke him.

The doctor on call was a beautiful African American woman, about ten years younger than me and clearly disapproving of the sport.

"He needs to wear headgear," the doctor said.

I know. I tell him all the time.

She had Weldon lie down on the table, and the nurse who always talked to me kindly when I came in with each of the boys spread paper toweling across his chest and neck and attached it to his T-shirt with a metal clip. She cleaned and then sponged the ear with iodine, injected anesthetic, and took a scalpel to the part of the inner cartilage swollen with blood, the hematoma that had developed under the skin. She was deliberate and calm, not speaking. Weldon sighed heavily. I was sure it really hurt. I was amazed at how much blood and fluid spilled onto the paper towels—it seemed like several ounces but was likely only one or two. All I could think was these poor, beautiful baby ears of his. Look what wrestling has done.

The only time he was ever in the hospital before was for these ears. At three, he had small plastic tubes surgically inserted in his Eustachian tubes to help avert his recurring ear infections. We were living in South Bend, Indiana, in a small rented ranch house I called the trailer home without the wheels. I remember how terrified I was as the attendants wheeled his small body into the operating room. He was all arms and legs then. Slender, with blonde hair and an energy that was unnerving; he was only gone a few hours and the operation was uneventful.

For months into years, he wore red plastic earplugs when swimming, and I was always careful washing his hair in the tub. At bath time I cupped one hand around each ear as I carefully poured water from a plastic cup over his head to rinse the suds from his scalp. I bathed him simultaneously in the tub with Brendan to save time, and Brendan would imitate me and cup his own hands over his ears. Brendan was a little more than a year old and would sit in the tub behind Weldon and splash and giggle until I washed his hair.

Like the doctor had promised, one day the tiny cylindrical tubes fell out and he had no more ear infections. He had outgrown them like so many pairs of his gym shoes and corduroy pants.

It was almost closing time at the emergency care center when the doctor wrapped Weldon's ear with a large bandage that made him look something like the illustration on the cover of *The Red Badge of Courage*. When he woke up in the morning, his ear was filled with fluid again, only this time it throbbed painfully. He was not happy.

Of course, it was my fault. I should never have taken him there. The doctor was an idiot, didn't know what she was doing. Why did I take him there? An assistant coach drained Peter's ear in his garage just a few days before. The garage.

After checking the instructions for a follow-up, I made an appointment with an ear, nose, and throat specialist. The office was in Berwyn and we had a 6:30 evening appointment the next day.

That day it snowed unforgivingly. I drove two hours in crawling traffic to get from my office to the high school to pick up Weldon, and another hour and a half to get a few miles to the new doctor's office. The windshield wipers were little protection against the driving snow.

"Why don't you just leave me alone?" He was shouting most of the way.

I was very upset and fought back tears. "I am only trying to do what is best for you."

We arrived before 8 PM, after I called the office repeatedly to beg for them to stay open. They did. This doctor was not so forgiving.

"You cannot wrestle with this ear for at least two weeks," he told Weldon.

Now I had done it. I had taken away his chance to win at wrestling, to place at state.

He fidgeted in the chair as the doctor told him he would drain it again and this time stitch it down—literally sewing the front of the ear to the back—so the ear would not fill up with fluid. The doctor told him wrestling was a dangerous sport.

"My son plays soccer, why not try that?" the doctor asked.

I didn't tell him Weldon already had. It was all wrestling all the time now, no more baseball, no more basketball, no more soccer. Wrestling was it.

When the doctor turned his back to Weldon and toward the tray of instruments, Weldon shot me a look that would melt many faint-hearted parents. I didn't care. I was going to fix what was wrong. I was not going to let my son have the ear. No matter how much he hated me at that moment, I felt I was right. I was going to fix this.

It was December and the season was heating up. Weldon said he had no choice; he had to compete. When I stopped Powell at a meet, frantic about Weldon's ear filling again with fluid, he told me not to worry, that it would be fine. Weldon did need to wrestle. He was fine.

This was crazy. He had an injury, for God's sake.

Almost a week after Weldon got the ear, after the trip to the emergency care and twice to the ear, nose, and throat specialist he despised, I e-mailed the boys' pediatrician, Dr. Sharon Flint. We developed a friendship over the years, seeing each other at the boys' annual physicals. We also attended the same church when I lived in Oak Park, our kids were roughly the same ages, and we went to some of the same parties. Our birthdays were a day apart, and we had breakfast to mark the occasion every year. I explained Weldon's condition to Sharon and she gave me the name of a specialist she recommended—Dr. Salil Doshi.

Weldon's ear hurt, he admitted reluctantly, and even with the stitching and the bandaging, it was filling up again. It did not look any better, even though now it was covered with dried, blood-soaked bandages. I was uneasy and wanted someone else to look at it. You had to take care of the ear within two weeks, get rid of the fluid, otherwise the ear would harden and would be completely deformed.

At his tidy office, Dr. Doshi listened to Weldon and nodded when Weldon explained how he needed to wrestle in a little more than a week. Finally, someone who understood him; I could read Weldon's relief on his face.

Dr. Doshi said an operation was necessary. It would be outpatient, but he would be under anesthetic. He would drain and scrape the ear and reform it as best he could, then he would stitch it, and it would return to normal in time. He was reassuring and confident. I made the arrangements.

A few days later, I was alone in the hospital waiting area, as I was always alone in the waiting rooms for the boys. I waited for their vaccinations, their dental cleanings, Brendan's orthodontic appointments, their haircuts, the parent-teacher conferences, for them to get showered and changed after games and meets. I waited for them in parking lots with the car running and the radio on, too tired to grade papers or return phone calls, just wishing I could go home or do something for myself, like go to the bathroom or shower.

It is what single parents do. You go alone to all the appointments, not making small talk or discussing the current crisis or conditions with a partner. You hand over the insurance card, write the check, answer the questions about history and immunizations, read the parenting magazines and occasionally the general interest magazine you would maybe buy for yourself if you had the time. You walk outside to make cell phone calls if you are not too worried, reschedule your meetings, rearrange your other children's schedules, scrawl notes on legal pads, check messages, make lists, wait for the prescriptions to be filled. You talk to yourself, you plan. You try not to waste the afternoon or the day. You are always the only one waiting, you are always the only one there, only sometimes wishing it didn't always have to be you. But you know it will always be you.

It was only a few hours of waiting for prep, surgery, and recovery this time, and now when they wheeled Weldon away on the table for the operation, he was almost six feet tall but still mostly arms and legs.

In the recovery area, the doctor spoke to me confidently and showed me Weldon's ear; it was perfect, pink, and well-formed, an exact match to his left ear. Hours later it would fill again and swell, but that would recede, Dr. Doshi promised. Less than a week later, Weldon wrestled in a match, his ear swathed in gauze bandages, his headgear secured with silver duct tape. He won the match. But he wrestled too soon; his ear did not have time to heal. He had the ear again. In spite of the operation and the drainings, he had the ear. When all the wrestling was over, after college, after it all, I told Weldon I was taking him back to Dr. Doshi and I was going to fix it.

Because that is what mothers do. I was going to fix it.

The following December, Brendan got the ear. He was wrestling junior varsity as a sophomore and apparently not wearing his headgear in practice either. As soon as I noticed it and Brendan confirmed it, we scheduled an appointment right away to see Dr. Doshi. His waiting room was crowded, a clientele of elderly, middle-aged, and very young. One was a beautiful teen who had multiple piercings on her ear, apparently infected. The nurses were kind and the magazines were decent—*National Geographic* and *Time*. I hated the waiting rooms with only golf magazines.

Brendan and I waited in one of the white-tiled patient rooms; Brendan reclined in the large leather chair that looked like a barber's chair. Dr. Doshi was pleasant and reassuring. After Weldon's visits and follow-ups, we were getting to be friends. This would go better than Weldon's ear did, Dr. Doshi said, since we didn't wait so long to come to him. Brendan winced when his ear was drained.

Unlike Weldon, Brendan agreed not to wrestle for a week to let it heal. So it did.

But in March of the next year, we were back. Dr. Doshi drained Brendan's ear again, puncturing the engorged ear with what looked like an X-ACTO knife, then a surge of blood, a few black stitches, and it was bandaged. We went home. But a year later, Brendan's ear appeared worse than Weldon's. Dr. Doshi said plastic surgery can fix the ears, not like new, but they could be improved.

Colin never got the ear, and I reminded him constantly to be sure he was wearing his headgear in practice. You would think wrestling made an athlete deaf as well. Colin said he didn't care; it would be OK, he would even like it if he got the ear. He called it a badge of honor. It made me incredibly upset, and I hoped he was not trying to make me upset, as sons sometimes do, just to temperature-check my reactions.

Because almost every time I look at Brendan and Weldon's ears, I feel like crying.

6

ALONE

1996–2010

had enough to do. I didn't need the scrutiny. For several years after my divorce in 1996, I did not introduce my sons to anyone I dated, mostly to save myself from the boys' interrogations and fears. First, I wanted to see if I even liked him enough to see him twice. Then, I could think about making introductions.

Raising the boys alone without financial assistance or physical reprieve kept me occupied, if not impatient. Meeting Mr. Wonderful was not the highest priority. In the time since my divorce, most of my first dates were coincidentally the last dates because I couldn't wait to get home and call a friend or one of my sisters to laugh.

"How often are your boys away for the whole weekend?" one date asked.

"Never." I noticed a perceptible shift in his demeanor.

The friend who fixed us up was apologetic when I told her on the phone.

There was the Italian accountant with the creaseless pants who asked early on our first date if I had my marriage annulled. He was

Catholic and wanted to remarry, and didn't see the point of going much further if I didn't conform to canon law.

Sure, some men were polite, attractive, and intelligent, but for years no sparks flew in my direction and no one was ever all that funny, interesting, or a better option than a hot bath, rented movie, or a stack of new magazines. I worked a lot—writing and teaching and giving seminars—and my kids were a lot. I didn't want to risk crying, feeling insecure, or having to tell my sons I met someone and had no idea what would happen. Mommy doesn't need a good time that badly. Dating strangers was scary—no sense risking ending up in pieces in the trunk of someone's car just because you wanted to wear pretty shoes out to dinner.

I understand I was afraid.

The boys didn't need any more surprises from a parent. I was predictable; I didn't bring home any threats to their homeland security. I also had hundreds of papers to grade, articles to file for magazines and newspapers, books to research and write. I had to give speeches, go to conferences and meetings. I had to make dinners. I had to make lunches. I had to make breakfasts. It was easier to go to bed early, wake up early, and get on with my day.

"He was so boring," I told Dana, my former college roommate, on the phone after a nice date with a nice man who was nice looking. "I think he went through his entire day minute by minute in chronological order."

"Oh, honey," Dana said. "They are all boring. You just forgot."

There were men I met in airports, on airplanes, or in shared cabs when I traveled for work. A man on a plane sitting in the row behind me and the boys—on our one and only trip to Disney World, because honest to God who in her right mind would go back—asked for my card and if I wanted to go out for a drink once back in Chicago.

"Mom, he's still smiling at you," Brendan said, his face contorted in complete disgust.

Some men who approached me were as old as my father would have been, and two were as young as thirty.

Most of the time I met them and that was it, no first or second dates, no phone chats, no follow-ups. Meeting someone was not difficult. Men talked to me in grocery stores. Not that I am all that flirty, but I answer them, even if I know the question about where are the sundried tomatoes is just a ruse. Still, meeting someone who was worth taking a risk on was nearly impossible. The idea of being close emotionally or physically with someone—anyone—was far too unsettling. I said no, thank you, to any offers but took the compliment they extended and that was all I needed for a while. It may seem as if there were a lot of opportunities, but spread them out over almost a decade and it worked out to twenty or so in about one hundred months, so not so many. Fewer than the number of phone solicitations in a year for aluminum siding, but more than your jackpot lottery win. I guess I could have taken a chance on one of them and fallen in love. But I dared not; the terrified of being fooled again thing.

I was realistic and knew my limits; I am not a woman all men find irresistible. But I do not hate any part of my body, because life was just too short for that brand of self-loathing, even if it was in jest. I want to be healthy and I consider myself attractive, but I do not obsess. I noticed that every year it took about ten more minutes of serious prep time to get to neutral, an additional fifteen minutes to appear as if I had a good night's sleep. Twenty more minutes on top of that to look good. An hour plus if the event was black tie and I had to do something inventive with my hair. Oh, and concealer, well, that's a given.

Years ago at a neighbor's cocktail party, I told the popular plastic surgeon who hosted Botox parties I was never invited to that I would prefer to be viewed in candlelight throughout my middle age rather than undergo any treatments that involved a knife or laser. I told him how I felt proud to be about much more than my looks, and that I was confident I was interesting and desirable without a breast job or eye lift or anything that would freeze my age lines with a poison ingested any other way could kill you. I also told him I did not want to have any surgery described as plastic. I wanted surgery that involved steel. He looked me up and down as if he was sizing up a horse he intended to buy.

"You can use some work," he said.

I didn't throw the drink at him. But in my fantasy it was red wine.

If I did go out, I was a good date. Polite, well-dressed, punctual. Didn't pick my teeth with a credit card—which I saw a woman do once at a friend's birthday party. I sat through a date's excruciatingly detailed stories of high school and college sports and asked appropriate questions. Smiled frequently.

I ordered the chicken—I always ordered the chicken. It was a lesson my brother Bill taught me when I was thirteen. I was getting ready for the homecoming dance my freshman year of high school in 1971. I wore a midnight blue jersey halter dress my grandmother made for me, and my hair was set tightly in the pink electric rollers with the steam. Bill walked by the room I shared with Madeleine with the green flowered bedspreads, a transition from the zebra print we had in an earlier phase. I was painstakingly applying blush and shimmer lip gloss in the mirror.

"Don't order the most expensive thing," Bill said. "Look at the price, don't get the steak." And then he went upstairs to his bedroom on the third floor, the one with the separate bathroom built for the servant couple who lived there with the original owners. We needed every room in the house for the eight of us, no servants.

Bill had his reasons for warning me. It was a cautionary dating tale in our house that his formal date his senior year of high school ordered lobster at a downtown restaurant. The young men at the table scraped together enough to pay his share of the bill, but barely. I was allergic to seafood, so I knew not to order that, aside from the price. The steak, no one had told me to avoid. This was practical, useful information, a major plus to having brothers. The next morning I proudly reported back to Bill about our meal at the revolving restaurant on the top floor of the Holiday Inn on Lake Shore Drive.

"I just ordered the house salad," I told him. "Nothing to drink, no dessert, no entrée. I think the house salad was about two dollars. Good, huh?"

He looked disappointed. "You should have ordered something. Guys don't like girls who don't eat."

I apparently exceeded the unspoken timetable for unattached healing when another calendar year would pass since my divorce and I was still available, on the market, my vacancy sign still flashing on the front lawn, still going to all-couples parties and black-tie events alone. Because no one had claimed me yet—and I had claimed no one for myself—it was as if I was doomed to rot, like a nectarine gone bad in the fruit bowl. I took offense at that, and sometimes said as much, when people would ask if I was seeing anyone. To everyone in the universe, being half a pair was a measure of my mental health and personal success.

"Are you remarried?" someone would ask as if we all were playing a matrimonial game of rock, paper, scissors.

I developed the pat answer that having a partner was not the measure of my well-being. I was well without one.

Staying out of the game was also about more than not wanting to waste my spare time. It was about my ability to trust someone, anyone outside my immediate family. When you get trampled, really trampled as I did in my marriage, it is not high on your to-do list to throw your heart into the center of U.S. Cellular Field or Yankee Stadium. I never understood people who had multiple marriages, one after the other, trading one in for the next like running shoes. They accumulated two, three, four spouses. Five even. I had a hard time talking to the same person on the phone two nights in a row.

I understand I have issues.

It was easier to be alone. It was cleaner, less dangerous, less fussy, and it definitely made me less insecure. No heartache. I spent so many years without romance, filling up my life with my children and my work and every detail to keep it all afloat, and my needs receded. It was not even noticeable at first; I stopped wanting and figured that wasting my time mourning the loss of real affection was like ranting at a sunset or a rainstorm. When you let go of the need, the need lets go of you.

Besides, I have had my heart broken open. So my heart opens only a little bit at a time.

Then in the summer of 2004, I suspended my fears and disbelief and waded slowly into a relationship with a man who was completely unlike my former husband. I regularly patted myself on the back for slowly falling—it was more like tipping or leaning—in love with a man who was kind, sensible, methodical, calm, and everything else my former husband was not. I loved him for who he was, but mostly for who he was not. And it was addictive, the feeling of being loved. I liked being able to relinquish control, even if just in the restaurant ordering wine. We were together for almost six years. It was great, until it wasn't. Nothing traumatic happened, it was just over; his choice.

But here is the thing, and here is what so many men miss. Women who are charged with doing it all—women like me who care for children and sometimes elderly parents and homes and careers— sometimes we want to do one less thing. Sometimes we do not want to be the only one to take out the garbage and drive to the store. Sometimes we are so tired of being together and in charge, we do not even want to talk, listen, or pick out a movie. Sometimes we would rather have a hot stone massage from a total stranger than a conversation of substance. Sometimes we want to melt quietly for a little bit before we go right back to being CEO of the family cor- poration. We don't want to be Super Woman all the time because it is tiring. So men need to know that we have to go back to that life, not pretend it does not exist. We just want a reprieve for a few hours. It's good if a nice, kind man is there too, one who reads a lot and can talk about the latest books. Not so good if he always acts like what I can give is never enough.

Many dates have told me I need to relax. Some have said I am an intellectual snob—I wasn't even trying that time my date said he had no idea what I was talking about, the references I made to stories, websites, events. Some say they can't keep up with me. Most say I am intense—the intensive care unit doctor for one, and I found that almost funny.

Here is what I want to tell any man who chides me for being too busy or too ambitious: I love what I do. I find exquisite meaning in writing things of topical importance, teaching young men and women to love a profession that I feel matters, mentoring adults and teens to find their voice and the need to contribute their ideas to a complicated world. I like standing up in front of an audience and telling stories. I like writing books. I like book signings and the line of people waiting to tell you that your words matter. I like learning, exploring, and discovering new ideas—feeling as if my time on the planet has meaning.

So there are times when it would be more romantic for you to pick up the prescriptions at the pharmacy because I don't have time to get them than for you to prepare a candlelit dinner for the two of us and ask me not to talk about what is going on in my head. To shush and be quiet. I want to listen to you, yes, I do, but I want you to listen back. Women like me will listen to you, honor you, but we can't take care of you. And I know how to nurture someone, yes, I know how to love someone well. I will do that for you. But please love me the way that I ask to be loved.

The problem is, no matter how much we say we are here for you, we can't be here for you only. We just can't. It's not a lie that we love you deeply and we do wish we could be yours alone, but we can't. There are other people we are in charge of, who have no one else.

We can pretend well enough in our lace dress with the Spanx underneath on a Saturday night to be sexy and carefree at the Brazilian restaurant that doesn't get moving until eleven or so, but it will be Sunday soon when we will have to go to Target to buy deodorant and peanut butter and poster boards. And then we will have to help with an English paper or a history project, and we can't tell you how much we desire you all the time because hot Beyoncé/Jay-Z desire is not something a single working mother can afford much of on a regular basis, especially when she is concerned about paying the mortgage and college tuition at this moment in time.

We hope you understand, but the truth is few do. Being in demand at work and home is not an aggressive act on my part. It is not at all about abandoning your needs. If it upsets you that much that I cannot sit in your den watching *CSI* every night, please go to the grocery store for ground sirloin, milk, and hamburger buns, and I will have an extra hour to spend with you and give you my full attention. I will watch *CSI*, but just one episode.

A romantic gift would be new tires for the car and an electrician to fix the kitchen light. For the past two decades, I didn't just need to forget my worries, I needed someone I trusted to talk out my next move at work, plan the book tour, the next website launch. I needed someone to help me navigate the teen years, and talk to three boy-men who sometimes were angry over everything, every day, all the time and I had no idea why. I needed someone to do more than just wait for me to stop talking so we could go to a concert. I needed someone to applaud my energy and not sigh with exasperation that I had a new project planned as soon as the current one was turned in. I would reciprocate, of course.

I would pitch in with his children and his work, listen, host dinner parties, plan anniversaries, spend time with his mother. Yes, yes. I would be Beyoncé hot when I could. But I would not be reprimanded for caring too much about my own children and caring too much about work. I care so much because I am the only one caring.

I can never stop being a mother of three sons, because that is who I am. I can put my cell phone on silent while we slow dance in the den, but I cannot turn it off. Not on the anniversary of our first date, and especially not on New Year's Eve. Because New Year's Eve could produce the apocalypse for teenage sons. I can take a long weekend, but I need to go home Sunday night because I have to throw in a load of laundry and drive someone to school from my own home the next morning. I do not want someone who is waiting for my ambition to subside and my children to get away from me. It is not that I do not know how to relax but that I never want to be great at relaxing. I have things to do.

In my case, I was the only one for my sons to call. There was no other parent. I always figured the boys would eventually move out of the house. I also figured I was worth the wait.

So for the last few years, since the end of that solid relationship, I have dated scores of men. Again, first dates mostly. Perhaps only three or four of these men did I go out with a second or third time, no one I trusted with my heart, goodness, even my home address. A friend recently said it is like the movie *50 Dresses*, except it is not all that funny.

The things I want to hear—and feel in my marrow—are not that I am irresistible in that light, but that I am understood. I need to be soothed with the notion that it will all be all right, all of it, not just tonight or this week. I want him to say that he knows I am afraid and not that he will rescue me, but that he will have my back, even if it only means he will answer his cell phone when I call as I am driving alone late at night and maybe get a flat tire. He does not have to solve my problems, but I want him to know I have them. I need him to understand you cannot say "forever" to a single mother a thousand times for years and years and hope she does not remember the promise.

I understand that some may say I am overzealous about my children, that I am distracted with all my work. But here is the bottom line: I do all of this because one of their parents left them on purpose. And that fact sears through me like a splash of acid. I know that in raising alone three boy-men, I get all the blame for everything they do or don't. I also know in my heart I get most of the credit. But I do what I do for them because it is what I need to do. It is just me holding the ball, me in the waiting room.

And I acknowledge it is a lot to ask. It will be until my youngest son graduates from college and moves out on his own, before I can spend more time with someone—for sleepovers, long weekends, and spontaneous trips to see the leaves change or the snow fall. But it really is only a few more years. And I will do what he needs and wants me to do to build something together that works for both of us.

Most men can't stand in line for five minutes for the perfect cup of coffee or wait patiently for a traffic light to move from red to green, much less come in third place after children and work. What I know is that at the end of my marriage almost two decades ago, I officially retired the notion of love as transformational tool, trying to get someone to do something or be what he is not. And I do not expect someone to change me. This is who I am. And I hope for someone I will love thoroughly and authentically who will believe that is enough. And he will love me for who I am in all my flawed imperfection.

It takes a long time to shape a human. It takes a very long time to shape three good men. And it takes more energy, focus, and commitment than I ever could explain to someone who does not want to hear, that this is the most important thing I will ever do. And it must be done. This is not elective. This is not a choice. And it can be done.

It takes help from family and friends and coaches who arrive in a high school wrestling room out of nowhere to be someone your sons will respect, love, and listen to. But you can't be drinking wine on somebody's porch when a son is in crisis. And you can't be whispering sweet nothings when a son is stranded and needs a ride home. Children can forgive many things—the hurts, the failures, the mistakes. But they cannot forgive you forgetting that they come first.

Buttons. That's what came to mind when I thought of having a partner, of being in love. In my mind's eye, I could see a huge drawer of spare buttons, some in the small plastic envelopes you get pinned to the sleeve of the slightly more expensive clothes, others just tossed in with excruciating randomness. I have a box of them at home in my sewing kit, hundreds of mismatched buttons: the gold military buttons and the flat pearlized ones in shell or tawny colors for blazers and jackets, the ones made of braided fabric, the small printed ones belonging to blouses or dresses I no longer own. All you want is two buttons that can hold together a piece of fabric for a good long time. You can spend a lifetime looking for another button similar to yours, simply trying to make somewhat of a match, just two together that appear to make a pair. You can expect symmetry—you can hope for it, pray for it, try to make two buttons work together—but no two ever match exactly, now do they?

7

GONE

2006

The screen message on my cell phone read UNKNOWN. I always answered anyway, no matter who it was, what time of day, or whether it was convenient: it could be an emergency for the boys. I once got a call when Colin suffered a concussion in seventh-grade gym class. Another time, I got a call when Brendan, in fourth grade at the time, landed on his knee on the playground and a wood chip daggered in so deeply it had to be removed in the emergency room. Weldon had the stomach flu one morning in middle school and needed to come home immediately. I answered that call too. I have turned around forty-five minutes into the hour-plus drive to work to retrieve a son, fix something, start over.

So I answered.

"Hello, Michele."

I had not heard my former husband's voice in about a year. His voice sounded as methodical and rehearsed as if it was delivered in a slow, intravenous drip. He said he was in town and wanted to talk to the boys and set up a time to see them. It was 2006, more than a year since he had seen them, more than two years since he moved to the Netherlands. I couldn't remember the last time he spoke to any of them.

"Call them yourself. They can arrange this for themselves," I told him. "They have the same e-mail they had before, the same cell phone numbers. We have the same home number."

We had a cordial conversation—brief and nonconfrontational. There was no point in confronting him. Attempting to redirect any of his behavior was like trying to sort through a tangle of live wires with wet hands. I hung up, slowed down the car, turned right off of Dempster Street at the next side street, pulled over to the curb, got out, and threw up. I stood in the street near a pile of leaves and breathed deeply until the nausea passed and I could get back in the car.

Later that night I told the boys at dinner. "Your dad called today to see when he could see you." I skipped the throwing up near the curb part.

Each son responded with a flurry of angry remarks.

When he entered their lives without preparation or warning, I felt as if we were all thrown into a Gopher Hunt arcade game at those manic kids' entertainment places like Chuck E. Cheese's. Plastic gophers pop up from holes on a flat board and the goal is to smack the gopher down with a rubber mallet; that's how the player earns points. Then another gopher and another pop up, over and over again, in different places each second without pattern or logic, until your time runs out and you put more tokens into the machine or walk away. And then? Nothing. As if the game was unplugged.

Two days later my former husband sent me an e-mail with the header DAD IS IN TOWN. The e-mail came as a surprise, like the phone call. In it he said he hoped the boys would call him on his cell phone. He also asked if he could have a private face-to-face conversation with me that would take fifteen minutes. He said he had an idea that talking to me would be "the first order of business in terms of reconnecting with the boys." And he signed it, "Love, Matthew."

His name was not Matthew. He changed it after he moved to Europe. Not legally, I gathered, since legal correspondence concerning him still listed his given name. Debt collectors called the house regularly asking for him by the name I knew.

The boys did not call him back. I would not meet him; I had learned from years of encounters with him that there was the lure, a promise of something, and then I surrendered my resistance, agreed to a meeting, and the trap snapped shut. He sprung on me a new hurt, a new demand, a new denial.

"Any ideas you have for me you can send in writing to me or my attorney," I told him in an e-mail.

My attorney had been trying to arrange a deposition with him for more than a year, and my former husband delayed the requests each time. He had filed a motion to stop all child support past, present, and future and would not show up for any deposition or court appearances. In the meantime, he paid nothing at all. For years. A deadbeat dad. Like in the movies. Like in the news stories.

Two more days passed and he sent another e-mail. He explained in the first few sentences that he would be busy celebrating the birthdays of his children from his second marriage, his daughter and her son. He did not mention that his son Weldon's birthday was also that same week.

In this e-mail he proposed that he and I write a book together on the "important message" of forgiveness, and said that he had already gathered his thoughts on the book. He went on to outline three "process premises": that our lives always reflect what we intend, that no one has ever treated us badly or wronged us, that every decision we make is the perfect decision at the time. He then elaborated with sixteen subpremises. He acknowledged that sometimes other people's decisions cause us pain, but it does not mean the decisions were not "excellent."

I was livid. Is genocide self-induced? Where does this put ethnic cleansing, violence, and abuse? A drive-by shooting, drownings? Were they all excellent decisions at the time, with no victim or perpetrator, just a reflection of what we truly want? Is everyone off the hook? Are you? Was being a father a part-time job you just quit? This psychobabble made me furious.

Of course, I would never tell the boys that his decision to have nothing to do with them emotionally, physically, or financially was an excellent decision. Never. No blame, no responsibility. No father should ever say that. No father should ever do what he did. I found the behavior reprehensible and immoral.

"I am busy with my own work, I will not write a book with you," I told him on the phone.

A few days later I picked up the package he sent to my post office box—a large document envelope with a photocopy of every card and love letter I sent him in our twelve-year relationship. I opened it and read them all. Some of them I distinctly remember writing and why—the birthdays, the anniversaries, the congratulations on this, the condolences on that. I suppose he intended for it all to soften me; the note he included said I once felt differently about him and here was the proof.

Yes, but he was a different person then. I didn't know he would disappear. I didn't know who he would become.

"Your father leaving has nothing to do with you," I said to the boys so often it made them mad. I wanted to be sure I said it, even if in some back room of their minds they did not believe it.

I no longer was angry at him for anything he did to me; that had dissipated years ago. I had worked hard to let it go. But our children are not adults. There is no mutual blame. These boys are your children. And you are the father. Every time I saw how the boys reacted to his omissions or his hurtful actions, every time they were reminded of his abandonment by his own sudden eruptions, I was infuriated for what he did to them anew. The fresh harm.

A good friend said his sudden departure to Europe gave the boys all the hurt of a parent's death with none of the insurance benefits. I was familiar with the insurance benefits.

"Do you have any other insurance? This has been canceled," the receptionist in the pediatrician's office said somewhat cheerfully when

I signed the boys in. I had three back-to-school physicals booked for the boys. They were eleven, nine, and six years old.

The receptionist called the insurance company again and handed me the phone. "This was canceled months ago by the policyholder," she told me.

My mouth went dry. The boys had been walking around—and wrestling—uninsured, even though the divorce decree included the stipulation that he carried the boys on his insurance. In the car on the way home, I called my brother Paul, and the next day he arranged to get the boys insurance before I could add them to mine. There was little at this point that my former husband could have done to reclaim the trust I had in him as a father. On a very basic level I did not trust he had their best interests at heart.

Part Two

TAKEDOWN

8

WAIT

October 27, 2006

"Dr. Werber saw your mammogram and wants you to come back as soon as you can for another look," her assistant said on the phone. I was in my office on campus and made an appointment for the following day, Friday.

You should know your life will change when the doctor calls you back in for a second, third, and fourth look. I had been going to Dr. Joan Werber for almost ten years for annual mammograms. Every year I was afraid to go, and every year they found nothing, the results were normal, I was fine.

Minutes after the return visit for the second ultrasound, I was in Dr. Werber's office. She shut the door.

"This is not good," she said, pointing to the X-rays and the ultrasound image she had tacked next to it. I had to push down the tears, swallow the suffocating fear. "We have to find out what this is."

She explained what would happen next. She was kind. She wrote her home phone and cell phone numbers on a card, then asked me what hospital I wanted to go to for the core biopsy. She got me in Monday morning with Dr. Kambiz Dowlat at Rush University Medical Center. The day before Halloween.

I couldn't shake the thought of how bad it would be for the boys if I died. It was too Dickensian. Their father runs away and has nothing to do with them. Their mother gets cancer. My boys should not be abandoned again.

Who would know them the way I do? Who would know they love the custard filling with fresh strawberries in their birthday cakes, the egg lemon soup from the Greek restaurant on 22nd Street? How they like drinking milk straight from the plastic jug and roast chicken stuffed with oranges.

I never should have grounded them; that would be all they remembered. Did I make their lives sing? I know I yelled too much. Sometimes I was mean. They did not understand me. So often I did not understand them fully. Did they know I loved them more than anything or anyone in the world? Was my part alone good enough to make up for the absence of their father? How would they be, who would they be, without either parent?

"I don't have time to die," I told my sister Madeleine when I called her.

"No, you don't. And I'll bring dinner. You don't have time to make that either."

I said nothing about my possible diagnosis to the boys over the weekend. Weldon was working on his early admissions application to one of the dozen colleges he was applying to for the following fall; it was due in a few days. He had to concentrate. I had to edit his final draft, and I knew he would be too worried or distracted if I told him or the other boys about the mammogram.

My doctor called me on my cell phone to see how I was. I was getting calls from my sisters and my brother Paul all weekend. I kept walking outside to talk, and saying everything was fine if the boys asked.

"What's the matter, Mom?" Weldon asked a dozen times from Friday to Sunday. "Why are you acting so weird?"

I was preoccupied, nervous, distant. I told him I was worried about work, making my book deadline, reworking the undergraduate curriculum for winter and spring, and a few upcoming speeches. I said I had a lot on my mind. I hated lying to him, but I knew he would worry if I didn't. Let him get the essay done; that was important. He asked me what seemed like every few hours.

I had to lie.

"Only you would have surgery at Bloomingdale's," Madeleine said.

Dr. Dowlat's office and the surgical center were in 900 N. Michigan Avenue in Chicago, the same building as the department store, as well as dozens of other upscale shops. The waiting area at his office was like the new South Loop restaurants with the single-syllable names—the adjectives like Red or East, where the waiters chatted in sweet tones and told you about the chanterelle mushrooms and the roux with leeks and garlic. Against the window were brown leather chairs and couches, burnt-orange textured pillows, large vases and sculptures. Smooth jazz played in the background. In the examination room, Dr. Dowlat calmly washed his hands. His face was oval with olive skin and thick black brows. His manner was regal, princely, and he asked me to lie down and pull down the top of the cotton gown. I was embarrassed, not anxious, to be bare-breasted in front of the doctor I'd just met.

The core biopsy procedure took a few minutes. It involved an extremely long needle and was only slightly painful, since he injected anesthesia into the area. I was eager to pull the gown back up. After I did, I dared to ask.

"In your experience, do you think this is cancer?" I was trying to sound nonchalant, as if it was just a small question, one he could answer off the cuff. I was a journalist after all; I was never one who could wait patiently for a test result or the answer to any question. I could take it, I needed to know.

"Yes, it is likely it is cancer," he said crisply.

The words hit like a fireball. In the same instant, both of his arms were outstretched, a father's instinct, and he hugged me briefly.

"I thought it was better to tell you than to have you wait," he said. "I thought you would want to know."

He told me what would happen next. I tried to take it all in but couldn't remember where I laid down my purse.

I did not feel the anger of *Why me?* Rather I felt, *Why not me?* I had seen a number of friends go through worse, from the death of a spouse to the death of a child. Years earlier when my brother Paul called to tell me his wife, Bernie, died in her sleep in their house in Florida, he sounded as if he was on helium.

"Bernie died," he said.

"What?"

And I had made him say it again.

Bernie had an undiagnosed brain tumor, and her death in 2003 left Paul and their three children steamrolled by grief. The next year, my sister Maureen's ex-husband died of a heart attack in his car. My friend, Norma, lost her only son, Ian, when he had a seizure at his high school, hours after she dropped him off with his backpack and a kiss. Both of my parents were dead. My brother Bill's wife, Madonna, was struggling with ovarian cancer.

People died. People who are not supposed to die, died. Just like that, driving to dinner, sleeping in bed, walking down the hall. Everyone died, but sometimes you had no warning and it made no sense. Not everyone was old. Not everyone expected it right then. Not everyone was prepared.

I have cancer.

"You get cancer from wearing deodorant," someone told me.

"I am glad for every sweaty day in the last thirty-five years that I wore deodorant," I told her.

You didn't know why you got cancer. Unless you were chain-smoking in an asbestos-battered building, eating chips of lead paint, and wearing moth balls around your neck, your guess was as good as anybody's. It was a complicated formula of genetics plus environment plus stress plus fate plus who knows what, maybe the perfume my mother wore when she was pregnant or the weed killer my father spread on the backyard lawn. It was the diet soda I drank. The milk I didn't. It wasn't the blueberries I ate or the red peppers I loved.

Cancer was everywhere. Everybody walked around with those pink ribbons on their lapels and the magnetized rubber versions on their cars. The good news was most of the time you got the breast cancer removed and you were fine. You couldn't start micromanaging and dissecting your history to single out every bit of everything you ingested or didn't ingest, because the figuring out would make you crazy. At first I couldn't even read the cancer websites. There were too many unhappy endings. Too many stories. Too much grief. Too many hypotheses. Too many women died.

Get it out of your body expeditiously, do what they say, have the treatments, take the drugs, and you'll be fine. You don't have to die. I couldn't die. The boys would have no one. I couldn't die now.

I went home and tried to act like nothing was wrong, but I couldn't sleep that night. I'm not proud of the way I told the boys the next day. The best explanation was that I was so exhausted from worrying that I cracked wide open like a barrel of red paintballs thrown against a white garage.

Halloween morning about 7:30 AM, I was taking Brendan and Weldon to their high school before going into work. I had known for sure for one day that I had cancer; it had been more than a week since it was suspected. I had said nothing to the boys about the diagnosis, acting as hard as I could as if nothing was the matter while inside I was a volcano of fear.

Brendan couldn't find his backpack and was throwing a fit.

"Mo-oo-om! Where did you put my backpack? I need my backpack! Mom!"

"Look in your room. Look under your bed. Look in the trunk of the car." I tried to breathe.

He kept shouting, swearing. It was several minutes before he found it. We got in the car and before I pulled out of the driveway, with Brendan still shouting, I did the unthinkable.

"Stop it! I have cancer!" I screamed.

"What did you say?" Weldon asked.

Then I started crying. And jabbering. "I found out yesterday, but I knew it could be a possibility," I wept. "You were right, something was wrong," I told Weldon.

As if by telling him I was validating his instincts and everything would be OK, he would be sympathetic now. As if I had not just scared the hell out of him.

The boys were quiet. I pulled out of the driveway and kept driving. I didn't have time to explain what was happening properly, and I am sure I would have if Brendan hadn't been so upset and if I'd had more sleep. I broke in a million pieces before their eyes. I told my friend Susy later that morning on the phone; she was my touchstone. Not only did Susy have two teenage boys, but she also had been the editor of a parenting magazine. Susy always had good advice on everything from sons to work to salads.

After a long pause, she said, "OK, so it's a Bad Mommy Moment. You get a few a lifetime."

What she didn't say was, optimally, you never had any.

"So then what? Did you drop them off and say, 'Have a nice day?'"

Pretty much.

On the bright side, this was not how I told Colin later that day. For him, I was saner. In the best of worlds, I wouldn't have screamed the news at the older two boys on the way to school. Like a lunatic, I made real all their fears about having no parents. I told Colin in a calm voice. You could say I was upbeat. Colin took the news well and I reassured him that I would be fine.

"My mom has cancer," Colin told Anne, Mike's mom, like he was saying I had brown eyes or a new pair of boots. Colin had gone to Mike's house in the next block to trick or treat. Anne called me as soon as the boys left.

"It's true," I told her.

"He seems OK with it," she said.

I hoped the other two would forgive me.

The surgery to remove the cancer in a simple lumpectomy was scheduled for the next week. All three of my sisters came at 6 AM to pick me up.

"I'll be fine," I said to the boys. "Go to school. You can call my cell at lunch. I'll be home when you come home from practice." The sitter would be there to make sure everything went on schedule.

I knew they would be watching me, and no matter what I felt like, I had to be positive, like this wasn't scary. Like I was not terrified that I was going to die and leave them alone.

Mothers die. Good mothers die.

A few minutes after I awoke in the recovery room following the surgery, Dr. Dowlat appeared. "You don't have cancer anymore. It's gone."

I liked that about him. Pragmatic, straightforward. I did not want to live my life counting down the days before it came back. Defining myself as a survivor one year out, two years out, three years out, every anniversary feeling terrified. I didn't want to think about cancer every time someone called to ask how I was. I told myself it was like having a flat tire. I got the tire fixed and was driving on, hitting the highway, moving ahead. I was done with having cancer. It was gone. I'd had a one-millimeter cancerous mass in my left breast, clean margins, no nodes involved. But it was the bad kind of cancer—as if there was a good kind—invasive.

"Let's plan something," I said to my sisters. My chest ached. I was so thirsty.

"Want to plan out a new kitchen?" Madeleine asked.

"That will make me depressed. I couldn't afford it."

We decided to plan a fiftieth birthday party for our brother Paul at the end of November. We picked a large Italian restaurant that could accommodate a crowd. Then we planned the menu for Christmas Eve, our family's traditional celebration, with gift exchanges between cousins, thirty-five of us in all. Maureen made a list of the twenty-one cousins to swap gifts. Every year I always asked to buy for girls; there were fourteen girls and seven boys in the cluster of nieces and nephews. I wanted a chance to buy something feminine and girlish, a reason to go to H&M, even if I did shop there for me and I was usually the oldest person in the store by three decades. I took the prescriptions for pain and infection, and we all went to the restaurant on the sixth floor of Bloomingdale's. It would be OK. I had plans.

9

BALLOON

November 2006

There it was, the perfect almond shape, like a ruby eye glistening wet and liquid, a glossy color you would paint a child's playroom. I stared at the shape in my left breast in the reflection of his wire-rimmed glasses, oddly unafraid, buoyed by a trusting detachment, as if it wasn't me I was watching, my body I was seeing. I was listening to the breath in my ears bouncing inside my head as if it was a favorite song on my iPod. It was a week later and this was the second step.

In the operating room Dr. Dowlat worked with nimble gloved fingers, red with my blood, his calm voice punctuating the silence with periodic reassurances. I was not asleep, I was not under, but I was dwelling in a suspended fiction, not quite sure how I could watch the image of my own operation without emotion. I was fascinated by the insertion of the brachytherapy tube, the new device that would deliver the radiation for my breast cancer treatment, the turkey baster that would save my life. I would have none of the skin problems or exhaustion associated with six weeks of traditional radiation. I would not get the tattoo. Every other external radiation patient I knew had a tattoo on her breast to mark the exact spot where radiation should be concentrated.

Dr. Dowlat described every motion aloud, into a tableside tape recorder to be transcribed for the surgeon's report, the one that would cost me twenty-seven dollars for a copy, the one I left unopened on my desk for weeks. I put it in the manila file folder marked *C*, next to the gas, electric, and Verizon wireless bills for four phones, one for me and three for the boys who didn't answer it when you needed them to. Maybe the folder would get lost and it would not be true anymore. I wouldn't have cancer. I dared not write out the full word on the folder for fear that labeling it would make it indelible, permanent.

The boys would find it cleaning out my desk after I was gone and they would cry. Here was the cancer file. Oh no. This was the beginning of the end. Mothers die.

Draped in a hospital gown with a floral print, my left breast exposed, seated upright at a seventy-degree angle, slightly reclined, I imagined that I looked like an old man watching the Super Bowl in a La-Z-Boy chair. I was not nervous, feeling only numbed pressure, no specific target points, even as the instruments went in deeper, inches inside my chest. It felt as dangerous as someone pressing against me on a crowded bus or the dentist working diligently on my novacained mouth. Dr. Dowlat quickly maneuvered the brachytherapy tube, implanting it in my chest, deep inside the hieroglyphic eye of blood, filling the attached balloon with saline. I took a breath and shut my eyes. But the image was still there.

He closed the single wound across the front of my breast. He had made a nick, a hole on the side of my body, like a bullet wound where they inserted the device. A catheter stuck out of my body about four inches, like a Bic pen. The nurse taped it down and bandaged the rest. The catheter would be where they inserted the radioactive pellet, and it would travel to the balloon that filled the cavity from the lumpectomy. My breast and side were sore. If this is what it took for implants, no thanks. I had briefly entertained the thought of having implants if I needed a mastectomy.

Maybe I would get stripper breasts.

I didn't need implants after all; they removed only the cancer in a neat slice and a tidy incision. I was a B cup before, so perhaps now I was a B–. And I didn't really want stripper breasts; I imagined they would bounce when I ran.

I tried to keep straight in my head the list of appointments, follow-ups, treatments, procedures, heartbreaks, terrors, details of what they all said, the what's nexts, the todays, the tomorrows. As if the mere chronicling of details would make it less terrifying, less like a bad dream.

The wound would need fresh dressing. I was to come back in two days to begin twice-daily radiation, Dr. Dowlat explained once we were back in his office.

"That's a lot of parking," I said.

"No one has ever remarked about the parking before," Dr. Dowlat said.

"Think about it, at least fifteen minutes of driving up the ramp to find a space and then you have to walk to radiation and then you have to pay at least five or ten dollars to park—twice a day. That would take so much time. It would cost so much. A week of that?"

Fay at the front desk explained I would get a parking pass to place on my windshield, park right in front of the building in the circular drive, and walk only a few feet to radiation.

I can park in front. I won't die.

The pink pamphlet I received with my diagnosis, "Breast Cancer Survivor Guide," had a self-described "patient-friendly" tone and stated: "Your diagnosis has probably put your emotions into a tailspin and your mind into overdrive. You're thinking: How will this illness disrupt my life? How will it impact my family? Above all, what are my chances of a cure?"

No, no chances, I had to be cured. I had sons. I had students to teach. I had a book coming out. This must be my cure. I had to be cured.

The pamphlet listed side effects. I half expected each paragraph to be punctuated with a smiley face. After diarrhea and constipation was listed "fuzzy thinking," defined as "symptoms dubbed 'chemo brain' include an inability to concentrate. You may also feel a bit 'down.'" Great, now I'll be dense and depressed; I'll forget what I am supposed to teach and I'll stand on stage in front of students for an hour and a half and whistle. Following the diagnosis of fuzzy thinking was the bold-faced solution in red. "Try to keep your perspective and sense of humor. If depression develops, talk with your doctor."

If it helped, I would laugh. I would heal by *Seinfeld*. I owned every season of the show on DVD. I loved the characters George and Elaine; Cosmo Kramer in smaller doses. The actress who played Elaine, Julia Louis-Dreyfus, was a few years behind me in college. She had been a star at Northwestern as well, in the campus productions, the comedies, the musicals. Her boyfriend, and later her husband, Brad Hall, lived across the hall from a man I dated in junior year. The sitcom dialogue made me laugh. I watched the DVDs for an hour or more a day.

Two weeks into my *Seinfeld* therapy, Michael Richards, the actor who played Kramer, made an explosively racist remark at a Los Angeles comedy club. The cringing scene was on YouTube and every news broadcast in the country. I couldn't watch anymore; suddenly *Seinfeld* episodes didn't seem so funny.

"Try *The Office*," a friend suggested.

I went online and bought seasons one and two of *The Office*, and at night I watched Michael and Dwight and Pam and Jim and laughed. I would get into bed and put a DVD in the player in my bedroom; the boys would come in and lie down near me on the bed or sit on the settee against the wall and we would all laugh. Sometimes I laughed so hard I would not think about cancer. And I could fall asleep. Colin would take off my glasses, place them on the side table, and turn off the television. And I would dream about Pam and Jim falling in love.

10

CLASS

November 2006

I wanted a new bag of ice to call my own.

At home we always had a few plastic food storage bags bulging with ice cubes shoved onto freezer shelves ready to be called into healing service. The boys used and reused the homemade ice packs for muscle injuries from practice, weight lifting, or a match. Lodged between Costco-sized sacks of pot stickers, or packages of ground turkey or boneless chicken breasts, they were on hand to soothe an athlete's aching body parts. I stopped endorsing the boys' practice of placing bags of frozen peas on sore muscles. Once I cooked a bag of frozen peas not realizing how many incarnations it had spent on Brendan's neck, Colin's shoulder, or Weldon's knee. Brendan recognized them right away.

"Those peas have been all over," he said when he saw them on his dinner plate.

"Rude, those are the ice pack peas," Colin announced.

"Did you use the edamame too?" I asked. Repulsed, I reached for a bag of salad to serve for dinner.

It was the day after the surgery to implant the brachytherapy tube, and I needed to attend a curriculum meeting on campus. I didn't feel so bad, I could go, I wanted to go. The journalism school was launching an ambitious multimedia initiative beginning with the freshmen with me as the lead instructor, overseeing a dozen instructors and two hundred students. The cancer just complicated everything, took time away from what I needed to do.

I was tired of thinking about myself. I wanted it all over and done. I wanted to get on with work, life, what the boys needed, and everything else. The work helped.

"How are you?" some people I knew not so well would ask, sometimes while standing in the deli line at Jewel, the local grocery store, their voice half-dipped in what felt like pity. Word got around fast in the suburb where we lived.

I minded that near-strangers would ask, perhaps to fill a gossip quotient, maybe idle chatter, or maybe they really did care.

I did not want to have cancer and I did not want to have had cancer, and I did not want everyone to ask me about cancer because I was sure I was OK. Yes, I was sure I was OK. And it was my breast, for goodness sake, not my big toe. Stop asking about my boob. Just a little cancer. I am Cancer Woman, no, Used to Have Cancer Woman. No More Cancer Woman. Wait, that sounds final. It was just a little, teeny eeny weeny cancer, the size of a thumbnail. Stage 1, not so bad. Invasive, that's not good, but stage 1, no nodes.

I didn't want anybody to know; yes, I was pretty sure I didn't want anybody to know. Then again maybe I wanted everybody to know so then maybe they could worry about it for me and I wouldn't have to.

Fireworks of pain shot through my left breast, and the left side under my arm was sore and swollen. Dr. Dowlat said it would hurt for a while and gave me painkillers I was afraid to take.

"Don't be a martyr," my brother-in-law Mike, who is a doctor, said. "If it hurts, take the pills."

I could keep going. I couldn't slow down. I kept working because if I didn't keep working it meant, well, it meant I was going to die.

Busy people didn't die. I had boys to raise, I had students to teach. The cancer was gone, I was dutifully doing everything they said to do. I would not die. I could not die. Sam I am. I am Sam. I was trying so hard to pretend it was all normal, while I was screaming on the inside that it was not. I couldn't concentrate for long stretches. Because over and over in my head like a mantra, I asked myself: *Where else is there cancer?*

In the hour ride to campus from my house, I kept the bag of ice on my breast—ten minutes on, ten minutes off; bag on at North Avenue, bag off at Cicero, bag on at the Edens Expressway, bag off at Dempster. It wasn't so bad with the ice. I listened to the Rolling Stones and tried to think about the new courses coming up and how they would work, how they had never been tried before at this level, and what I needed to get done before January.

Mick Jagger was an old man and he was still rocking. Keith Richards might live forever.

That first week of the winter quarter I would stand in the lecture hall with all new material. I would stand there with my tamoxifen-generated mood swings and hot flashes, a hole in my chest where the cancer used to be and a closed, bullet-hole scar where the radiation tube had been, pretending everything was dandy. Cancer was one thing. Teaching alone unprepared before two hundred eighteen-year-olds for an hour and a half in a mandatory class was quite another.

I felt as if I was swimming in glue.

"I don't feel like myself," I told Colin later.

"Who do you feel like?" he asked.

I didn't have an answer.

My shapeless, dark-colored sweater concealed the bag with enough ice to cool a very small keg. But it was starting to leak. Just before I walked into the faculty conference room, I took the ice off. I later placed it on the floor beside my chair; I could excuse myself in case the pain increased and stick it under my sweater.

When I walked into the room, five of my colleagues applauded. It was OK they knew; I was grateful.

"This is the first time in a month I have been to a meeting where I kept my shirt on," I said. I knew as soon as it came out of my mouth it was a dumb thing to say.

But when you have cancer—and I imagine most any other disease as well—the separation of the personal sphere from the medical arena involves such a pervasive and thorough disruption of your privacy, you get confused. Mostly it's because you feel as if you are evicted from your own life.

You initially were red-faced and embarrassed when someone new saw you half-naked in the offices of the oncologist, surgeon, or radiologist. But after you did it so often you expected to be topless in front of every person you met. *Nice to meet you, want to take a peek?*

"So you teach journalism?" the resident asked the first time I met him after radiation. He was trying to make small talk, I gather practicing his bedside manner on topless cancer patients. "My roommate just graduated from there in the master's program."

"What's his name?" I asked, pretending this wasn't incredibly awkward.

He told me. I knew him. He would go home that night and tell his friend about Professor Weldon's breasts.

I began teaching journalism as an adjunct ten years earlier when I was freshly divorced. I had a cinematically romantic notion of what it meant to be a college professor. I thought the whole scenario would resemble *Goodbye Mr. Chips*, *Wonder Boys*, or even *Dead Poets Society*. I would engage impossibly bright, grateful, and eager students who would hang on my every syllable, taking notes on all my comments and nodding in agreement, calling their parents to remark on my brilliance and insight and how grateful they were to be in my class. They would quote me years later when they won awards. They would all like me.

When Julia Roberts played a college professor in *Mona Lisa Smile*, I thought, *there, that could be me*. Every part of my life was mimicked in at least one scene of every Julia Roberts movie, and most of them have happy endings. You befriended your students who emulated you and whom you inspired to achieve greatness; that was rewarding. You could do all that while looking amazing. And when the spring quarter of the school year was over, I would relax all summer, doing something intellectually stimulating that would further my career. Write more books and articles, give more speeches. Then in September, I would do it all over again. I wouldn't ever burn out. I would never have a bad day.

It wasn't exactly like that. No, really not at all.

I saw myself in the young women who sought my advice and I saw my sons in the young men who asked for recommendations and sometimes told me jokes after class. I expected to connect to them all in a way that rewarded us both because I liked them all even before I met them, just by seeing their fresh names full of possibility on the roster, their photographs so innocent and promising. Every quarter I was determined to make this their favorite class ever, align myself with their trajectories, guarantee their successes, show them what I knew, help them every way I could. Help them meet their goals, their dreams. Be their Julia Roberts.

Teaching was more work than I imagined in my fantasy, definitely more work than I had done in a magazine or newspaper newsroom or as a freelancer juggling magazine, newspaper, and any other writing and speaking assignments I could land. For every one hour of lecture, I could do at least ten and more likely twenty hours of preparation. Most of the faculty did that. Aside from the hours of research for every class, it was the grading that could do you in, six or more hours a day to edit lab and homework assignments—and the scores of hourly e-mails that demanded immediate action. The committee meetings, the advising sessions, the faculty meetings, the mandatory meetings when someone of note or newsworthiness came to campus, the lunches in the dean's office with the same sandwiches every time, the favors from colleagues in other parts of the university, the feedback sessions, the lectures of friends, the lectures of visiting authors, the announcement of new procedures, the announcements of ended traditions. There was a parade of new deans—more than a half dozen over the years, each one with his (always his) agenda and peccadilloes, favorites, and danger zones. New turf to navigate. New rules to ingest and obey.

There were the colleagues you shared birthdays with and the secretaries who made you laugh and brought you Christmas gifts. There were also colleagues who did not respond when you said hello in the hall. Colleagues in meetings who countered whatever you said.

And there were the course and teacher evaluations filled out online that included, "I hate her chunky bracelets," "Her voice is annoying in the morning," and my all-time favorite, "She teaches us too much." Of course many of the comments were gratifying, but there were always hate-filled comments about what I wore, my feminism, or that I should be despised because I had age spots on my face.

Still, it was an undeniably good gig. Teaching at what we considered the best journalism school in the country at one of the top universities in the world. Great benefits. Retirement plan. Dental! Vision! View of the lake from the parking garage and the classrooms in the buildings where I taught. Coffee in the faculty lounge. Smart women friends. Big ideas, always talking about big ideas to change the world. A top administration that felt open and warm and encouraging. Professors and adjuncts and researchers you met at cross-disciplinary functions who were blindingly bright and also trying to manage their roles in the universe.

And for your part in the whole equation, you did what was asked, you did what was expected. You never said no. You contemplated what new, inspiring lesson to teach every second, how to improve your approach, and you stayed awake nights thinking about how to help improve students' writing and reporting, what you could do or say to make it go well.

You ignored the white-haired male colleagues who snored or snarled in faculty meetings—and that was definitely the majority—who objected to every new idea, even the name change for the school. And you ignored the mean woman who smirked when you commented in a meeting. It was OK because you were smart enough to sit near the people you liked in the group meetings and the convocations and the lunches and the presentations, the people like you who worked hard and cared about the students and the quality of the content, the journalists who were still committing journalism, not just talking about it, the ones with the book deals, the documentaries in the works, the new sites, the side gigs, and the excitement about all that was new in media and the world. There were enough of them to make it fun.

I learned that some quarters the teaching was more difficult than others, and that most times I could divide a large lecture class into thirds. All the students were very intelligent; it was the attitudes and approaches that varied widely along this triptych.

A third of the students were every professor's dream—ambitious, polite, energetic, eager, respectful, very advanced in their skills and abilities. Another third were ambitious and respectful, newly exposed to the skills needed, but eager to learn. Another third were what academics call strategic learners, who cared principally about the grade and what it took to get the grade they wanted. Some students would come to my office and argue over a single point on a grammar or current events quiz, even though it was one point out of four hundred possible points in the course. We would go over the student's concerns, I would show him or her the page number of the correct answer, and the student would still ask for credit. These students, at any given moment, any hour of any day, wanted an answer right now, right *now*, even if they e-mailed me at 3 AM on a Tuesday.

"You never answer me until Sunday when I e-mail you on Saturday, and I do my homework on Saturday," one student chastised me in an e-mail. Another told me in an e-mail the quiz was too "fucking hard."

It struck me as odd that it never occurred to some students that a professor would have a life, his or her own children, problems, concerns—heck, cancer. That sometimes we walked up to the podium out of a complicated life.

Sure, most were not that way. Many more students from India to Indiana made me want to call their parents and say what a good job they did raising smart, curious, and respectful people with ambition, talent, and humility. I got to do that at graduation—meet their parents—and promised to stay in touch while they took pictures of me with their children on their digital cameras under the white tents that housed enormous strawberries, the red punch, and the small cucumber-and-turkey sandwiches. With many of the students I felt deeply responsible for their initiation into the profession, for helping them love storytelling, for helping them become writers. They hugged me at the start of every quarter, brought me small gifts, mementos from a study abroad quarter.

There were former students from as far back as my first year of teaching who called and e-mailed me with news of new jobs, new accomplishments, awards, life events, even heartaches. A few invited me to their weddings. To be electively included in their circle of friends and mentors was an honor, because that was their choice. They did not have a choice in choosing me as their professor; I taught the "vegetable classes," the required fundamental skills classes in their major, not the "cake" classes of the electives with ten or sixteen upper graduate students, the seminars, the independent studies. But for some of them, after they finished the course, years later, they did choose me.

The truth is, it is a lot of fun to stand in front of a group of students and talk about ideas and to get them to talk back, engage, and demonstrate what they learn. And to do it at a university you respect and feel loyalty to—real loyalty, not just *I am here for the time being* loyalty, but a place you care about deeply. And it is rewarding to feel for about ten seconds at a time that you are Julia Roberts, even if you have chunky bracelets some hate and age spots you yourself are not so particularly fond of, right there on your face for everyone to see.

■ 11 ■

RADIATION

November 2006

"You have beautiful hair," she said when I took off my hat and placed my purse and briefcase on a couch near her in the waiting area. I hung up my coat and stuffed my hat and scarf in one sleeve. "I lost all my hair," she explained and gestured to her paisley headscarf.

"I like your scarf," I said.

"Today is my birthday. I'm seventy-six."

"Happy birthday." *I want to be seventy-six.* I didn't know if I should keep talking or ask more questions. I wasn't sure exactly what radiation treatment waiting room protocol was.

Should we all exchange cancer stories, prognoses, recurrence likelihood percentages? Are cancer jokes OK? Is this where we cheer each other loudly or silently pretend everyone in the room is not obsessed with measuring the odds?

This was my first time. But it already felt different than a regular doctor's office; more like a block party without the cocktails and food. At the front desk the staff was remarkably effusive, as if they were greeters at a health club or Walmart, smiling as they checked off your name and handed you a parking pass to put on your dashboard so you could park close to the automatic sliding door off the circular drive. No one was ever in a bad mood here; they were on the safe side of cancer.

A dozen or so other patients looked up from crossword puzzles or magazines and away from the morning show on the mounted television and wished her a happy birthday. A man in his sixties or seventies, neatly dressed in dark pants and a cardigan sweater, strolled in, stood in the center of the room with his back to the flat-screen TV, waved a broad sweep of hello, and boomed, "Good morning, how is everyone today?" as if he was Norm and this was the bar in *Cheers*.

"Good, great," was the chorus's response. No one replied, "OK, except for the cancer."

He hung up his gray parka, poured black coffee into a Styrofoam cup, and helped himself to two of the sugar cookies in an open tin before sitting down with the newspaper he carried under his arm.

The waiting area was the size of a motel lobby, the sort of motel you stay in for just one night for a business meeting or a stopover on a long drive to somewhere else, a sixty-nine-dollar-a-night spot you see in the Midwest with the packaged dairy creamer and no wireless connections. The coffeemaker was always on and a microwave sat beside stacks of brochures for local water parks, ranches with hourly horseback riding lessons, antique shops, and wax museums.

I was the youngest person in the waiting room that morning, but still much older than the medical residents who walked briskly in and out of the room, their white lab coats crisp, their hands in their pockets, their expressions pensive.

"Jeez, some of these people look really sick," Paul whispered to me. He had picked me up for my first morning radiation treatment. "You look pretty good in comparison."

This building in the massive hospital complex was called the Woman's Board Cancer Treatment Center and thankfully not Outpatient Center/Nuclear Medicine, where I had gone for an earlier test. *Nuclear* was not an adjective you want in any part of your medical treatment. I remembered the news stories in 1979 of Love

Canal and saw *Silkwood* twice, mostly because I couldn't believe Cher could actually act. This radiation was serious business; only a week earlier news reports announced that Alexander Litvinenko, the former member of the Russian Federal Security Service, had died with the diagnosis of "acute radiation syndrome," a deliberate poisoning from polonium-210. I was almost positive I was not getting polonium. Palladium was what I was getting; that was different.

At Dr. Dowlat's suggestion, I would be having internal radiation at 9:50 in the morning and 4:30 in the afternoon every day for five days, compared to traditional external radiation therapy once daily for six to seven weeks; that burned your skin. Internal radiation treatments needed to be six to seven hours apart; staff gave those morning and late-afternoon times to accommodate patients who were working. That way we could work between treatments.

The senior director of the undergraduate program got me an office to work in at the university's downtown law school and continuing studies campus in between treatments. That way I would not have to drive from treatment on the near South Side all the way up north and back—about fifteen miles each way.

She got me space in a lecturer's office with a radiator that hissed aggressively and a view of the lake if you strained your neck. I drove there after the morning session, parked in the Neiman Marcus building, and walked through the first floor, spraying samples of delicious perfumes on my arms and neck.

I was thinking maybe it would be nice to go home and lie down in between treatments, but maybe the senior director was right—it was better to be busy. I did have to work on the curriculum.

The kind of radiation I was having, internal brachytherapy, had only been available after FDA approval for breast cancer treatment for four years. More than thirty thousand breast cancer patients had had this form of radiation, one of the pamphlets read, this one with a large pink tulip on the cover as if it was an ad for Miracle-Gro. The brochure resembled the flyer I got in middle school health class on menstruation, making the process seem so feminine and pretty and benign.

Thirty thousand people with this kind of radiation. Not so many when you consider that was about half of the number of fans who went to any single Chicago Bears football game in Soldier Field, the smallest stadium in the NFL. More than twice as many people lived in Oak Park.

The brochure did not mention that the total bill at the end of treatment would be more than $90,000 for radiation alone. Insurance covered most of the bill. Thank God and the university for good insurance. The brochure also did not mention what the radiologist told me in person.

"You should not be around pets or small children during the days of treatment," said Dr. Adam Dickler, my radiation oncologist.

What?

"Just a precaution," he said.

"How small of children?" I asked, knowing my boys at ages twelve, fifteen, and seventeen were probably in the "big" category.

"Newborns or infants, babies," he answered. "Your boys are OK."

Did the radioactive material seep out of me after the treatment?

I remembered the first *X-Men* movie where Anna Paquin played a superheroine named Rogue whose mere touch killed people. And then there was *The China Syndrome* with Faye Dunaway, back when Jack Nicholson was not so old and creepy—oh, so many movies where people died from the radioactive material. So what would happen in five, ten, fifteen years to us, the ones who opted for this kind of radiation? I didn't want to dwell on the possibility that this treatment was experimental. I read *Flowers for Algernon* as a kid and saw the movie *Charly*. He was part of an experiment and he died. The *New York Times* later ran a front-page story on the experimental treatment. It sat on my desk for days until I had the nerve to read it all the way through.

Dr. Dowlat endorsed this course of treatment emphatically. On my next visit I asked him about the article.

"It is not experimental," he said. "It is effective."

I trusted him, I had to.

Down one hallway, nurses escorted patients who were receiving traditional radiation, the external X-rays, to an area where patients changed into hospital gowns and radiation was aimed at their cancer site, a spot tattooed in their skin. Everyone else in the waiting room was getting this kind; their names were called every few minutes. For the internal radiation, I went down another hallway and I was the only patient there.

Isn't anyone else having this kind? Hello?

A nurse about my age, with a round, pleasant face and reddish-blonde hair to her shoulders, called my name. We went into a patient room where she checked my vital signs and the wound site. She asked me questions and made small talk; we both had sons named Brendan, the same age. She had a daughter, younger than her son. Next I would be going to another area for the radiation.

"Can I read a book?" I asked her.

"It's only ten minutes. Why not just relax?"

Sure, I can relax while the deadly radiation is inside my body. Sure. Might as well knit a sweater.

Dr. Dickler directed me to still another room where he told me to lie down on the metal table. I did not need a hospital gown. I wore a shirt that could be lifted up easily. He would insert the tube to deliver the radiation into the catheter that was sticking out of my body like a throwaway pen. I liked Dr. Dickler; he was very friendly, personable. He looked way younger than me. Everyone on this side of the cancer was way younger than me. Except Dr. Dowlat.

Signs on the door, in the hallway, and on the walls were in bold black letters: DANGER. RADIOACTIVE. DANGER. The round sign had the three-winged symbol for radiation that looked like a kitchen fan. DANGER. I get it: radioactive.

The flat table had a foam pillow for my head. Dr. Dickler connected my catheter to the machine that would deliver the radioactive pellet, the size of a grain of rice, he explained. The pellet was smaller than the cancer Dr. Dowlat excised. I would be alone in the room while the radioactive seed was inside my body. Dr. Dickler would watch me from another room and he could hear me at any time, he said. I could ask questions, I could speak to him and the technicians monitoring the treatment.

One of the technicians looked like a character in a Dr. Seuss book with a gentle face and a white bushy mustache. Posters of forest scenes were taped to one wall of the laboratory, which was about the size of my living room. My dentist has posters taped to the ceiling as well, but he also has a chair with a remote that controls heat and massage, really just a vibrating bump that moves from shoulder to knees. And your mouth still hurts.

Dr. Dickler flipped on the machine, left quickly, and the door clicked shut. The machine that delivered the radiation looked like R2-D2 in *Star Wars*; it was the size of a shop vac. Looked harmless enough, except it wasn't. DANGER. RADIOACTIVE. DANGER. It was like a scene in an early Woody Allen movie. Prime time for a panic attack, and I was trying not to have one.

"We can hear you in the observation room if you need us," Dr. Dickler said.

Don't worry, you'll be just dandy here with the deadly radioactive material in your chest. No, you stay, just let me get the hell out of here.

Alone on the table, I couldn't feel anything going into my body, but I could hear the clicking and whirring of the machine like an electric toothbrush. I tried to relax, picturing the radioactive pellet sitting inside my chest obliterating the cancer site.

Was it glowing? Was this my kryptonite? If this is so fine, why did all the doctors and technicians run away as soon as they connected the catheter and flipped the switch? Breathe. Stop thinking. Relax. I'll pretend I'm getting a pedicure, or a massage. That's it, I'm at the spa. I could pretend I'm at Miraval and waiting for the masseuse to find the hot oil to rub on my legs. This isn't so bad. But it is quiet, completely quiet, deathly quiet except for the whirring. They should have music piped in, not the wind chiming, wave-rushing relaxation soundtrack played in every spa in every hotel I have ever visited, but maybe a little Motown, some Sheryl Crow, what the heck, Melissa Etheridge—the Cancer Singers. What's that smell? Is that burning? Did they give me too much? Am I on fire?

"Something smells burning," I said out loud, motionless on the table. "Is that me?"

"Nothing is burning, it's fine, you are not burning," Dr. Dickler answered from behind a glass wall, just as he said he would be able to. "Just a few more minutes."

I pictured myself cooking from the inside out, like one of those soy burgers in the microwave that did not taste at all like real meat but were only 120 calories. For ten minutes, ten long minutes, this was good. I would do whatever they said. I would take whatever form of therapy they suggested. I would eat it, I would drink it, I would let it sit in my body, I would wear it. I would agree to it all, I would not fight, I would not argue, I would do it. Because the alternative was far worse. My friend Lisa lost a close friend to breast cancer when we first met. Her friend decided she did not want to do the radiation and the chemotherapy. She did not want to go through it all; instead she chose alternative approaches, herbals and teas and acupuncture. She died and she had children.

Yes, I was scared to die. For the record? I was afraid to die because of my sons.

When I thought about dying, I really did not think about me. No really, I did not. I was not scared for me, not that I was ready for it or anything. I was scared for my boys. Probably since my thirties, after my father died in 1988, I began to feel this low-pitched drumbeat urgency that this was all there was and I was close to the halfway mark. When my mother died in 2002 she was graceful, had dignity, was unafraid. And it secured my feeling that this was finite, but that it was OK. All of my mother's children were grown—we were fine, taken care of, on our own. She seemed at peace.

Because of all of that, I have felt as if I was renting space in the world, had squatter's rights. I knew none of this here was permanent, knew I wasn't permanent, knew there was no overtime. I absolutely had better give this my all. Work hard, do all I can, love my children as much as I can, give back to the world. Don't relax. Work, accomplish, keep going, say what you mean. Mean what you say. Push for the next project, try to write another book as soon as possible. Be heard. Be good to my family. Be kind to my friends and plenty of strangers. Make a difference somewhere that adds to the cumulative joy of someone. Try. I didn't own the place, no guarantees. But I didn't want it to be my time to go just yet.

Time was up. It did go quickly; it was only ten minutes. Twenty minutes a day, one hundred minutes total. Not bad if one hundred minutes can add years to your life, and that was what they promised. That was what I banked on. I said thank you to Dr. Dickler after he removed the long tube from my catheter. I went back into the patient room, and the nurse with the son named Brendan changed my bandage and told me she would see me later in the afternoon.

This time I would bring cookies. That would be nice. Be the patient who brought food. When I saw her later she commented on how nice I looked and complimented me on my shoes or my skirt or my jacket. And everyone on the safe side of cancer smiled at me and was pleasant. And why not? They didn't have cancer. The rest of us did.

"No need to come back with me, I'm good," I told Paul.

"Sure, OK," he said.

But I knew he would show up, if not tomorrow then Friday. And he did show up, twice more that week; I walked in and there he was in the waiting room. My sister Maureen came once as well.

When Paul came to the hospital, we talked and he told me jokes. Paul and I were close mostly because we were just a year and a half apart. I fixed him up on dates in high school, college, and after college. He fixed me up for high school and college formals, and all of them I forgave him for and he forgave me. He was my closest friend. When I was first divorced, he and his wife, Bernie, invited the boys and me over for dinner a lot. We went out to eat often, even vacationed with Bernie and their three. He included me in dinners, parties, and all-couples events and never once made me feel awkward that I was alone. He had a book signing party for my first book, selling copies in his backyard. He had been a champion for the boys and went to their wrestling meets and football games and was always there for us. Since his wife died—"passed" Paul said because I don't think he could say "died"—we talked almost every day, sometimes more than once. "U.P." my boys called him, for Uncle Paul. When I got home after the second round of radiation, I told the boys U.P. was there.

"That's good, Mom. It's good you have U.P.," Brendan said.

When I started radiation, Paul lent us his Nissan Altima so Weldon could drive himself and Brendan to weights at 5:30 AM and I could sleep another hour before getting up to get Colin ready and get to work myself. Weldon also needed the car to drive to wrestling camp at 5 PM. With one car, that was impossible. I did it one day, raced home from work in an hour, picked up Weldon, drove the hour back, did work in the car while he was at practice, then came back home. That was exhausting, plus a total of five hours in the car for the day. Paul's generosity was enormously helpful. After a few months, he surprised me with the title to the car; I had thought it was a temporary loan until I had my strength back.

"It makes me feel good to help you," Paul said. "I promised Mom I would."

■ 12 ■

POISON

January 2007

The young woman at the reception desk with the gold bangle bracelets was chirpy. The chairs against the wall were filled with patients. It was my first appointment with the oncologist on the eighth-floor Radiation Oncology Center.

"Do you have a copy of your last will and testament?" she asked.

"What did you say?"

"If you don't have it, that's fine. Do you have your insurance card with you?"

Still numbed from the first question, I fumbled through my purse to find my white insurance card and handed it to her. She continued to process my information, printed out a wristband, attached it to my left wrist, and then handed me my paperwork.

I was positive she just asked me for a copy of my will. A nurse, doctor, or administrative assistant has never asked me for a copy of my will; not for my emergency appendectomy, the births of my three children, the wisdom teeth extraction when I was twenty-one, even the lumpectomy I just had. Old, sick people need copies of their will when they go to the doctor. I was only forty-eight. And I had cancer. *Had*. Past tense. I did not have cancer anymore.

"I'm not planning on dying today, so why do you need to have my last will and testament before I meet the doctor?"

"We just want it on file."

Got cancer? Everyone got right to the point. I was grateful she didn't ask me if I want to be cremated. If anyone did ask, the answer was no. I would prefer the traditional route, the elaborate casket, the wake from 3 to 9 on two days, not just one, where hopefully the boys would be on time, have neatly pressed shirts, and not chew gum. The funeral could be first thing in the morning, a traditional mass with pretty music, my niece Alyssa could sing, then a printed program done on InDesign, not just thrown together, with hopefully a good picture of me, one where I am laughing maybe and my hair looks good. I hoped Madeleine would help the boys with their eulogies. God knows what they would say. Oh, and no elaborate headstone. I found those obnoxious—the huge statues of angels, the gilded and marble tributes, what was the point. I didn't visit my mother and father's graves, though all my brothers and sisters did. Not out of disrespect, of course; I really didn't want to. It didn't make me feel better; it made me feel worse. I didn't need to go to their graves to talk to my parents. I would tell the boys they didn't have to visit my grave, but I would not bring that up now. That wouldn't be for a very long time. They probably wouldn't visit anyway, so it would be better if eventually I told them I didn't want them to, then they wouldn't feel any pressure. But I would be old when that happened. I would be ninety, maybe one hundred. I would get very old. *Why did she need the will today? I was not going to die today.*

Mike offered to drive me and waited there if I needed him to talk to the doctor; sometimes the doctors spoke in codes. I considered myself an educated person, and I took four years of Latin in high school, but some of the words the doctors said I had never heard before. Like *brachytherapy* and the drug names. I knew the basics: penicillin, the sulfa drugs the boys have taken for infections, and the drugs my mother took in the last years of her life—Fosamax,

Halcion, and a half dozen more. They could just as easily have been the names of cars.

The waiting room was filled with close to one hundred people waiting for several doctors in the center. Many were older people, some younger, some more were bald. People in wheelchairs, people with walkers, men, women, white, black, Asian, Hispanic—reading the paper, the magazines, drinking coffee, watching TV, staring straight ahead. It was like a gate in the airport terminal, but with oxygen tanks. Like every other element of synchronicity, you got a diagnosis of cancer and suddenly the whole world had cancer. Molly Ivins had cancer. An outspoken newspaper columnist and author, I saw her speak at a conference a few months ago; she was thin and looked weak, but her words could still knock over a charging bull. We both worked at the *Dallas Times Herald* in the 1980s, and when she was in the newsroom, boy, everyone knew it. She died. Lots of people with cancer died.

"I like your skirt," a woman in a turban said as she smiled to me.

You could gather a lot of compliments in the radiation and oncology waiting rooms, I have found; polite consideration, everyday niceties, warm greetings, kind encounters are the norm. It was as if you arrived in this place after your diagnosis and we all figured life was too short, so why the hell not, might as well be as pleasant as possible; we were all in the same boat.

"Thank you," I said. "I like your blouse."

Mike and I moved from the reception hall to sit in another crowded area; a few minutes later, a nurse called my name. She was also smiling and bubbly, like a human fruit smoothie.

"I can't wait to get away this weekend," she told me in a familiar tone, like this was not the first time she weighed me or met me, but we were old school friends. For a second I forgot where I was; it felt like she and I could talk about shoes. Or the weather, or what we each had for dinner the night before. She weighed me, took my blood pressure, and walked me back to a treatment room where I would meet Dr. Ruta Rao. In oncology centers, losing weight is a bad thing. They want your weight to stay the same. I could have started to hyperventilate. But I kept breathing slowly, through my nose.

Like most every doctor on my support team but my surgeon, Dr. Rao was younger than I was. She was beautiful and petite, polite and soft-spoken. After some small talk, she handed me a printout from Adjuvant! Online. I was not sure why it had an exclamation point in the title; I guess they really mean it.

Don't use exclamation points in your writing, I told my students. Save that punctuation to follow the words fire *and* help.

On the left-hand side of the single white sheet were boxes the doctor had typed in under the heading PATIENT INFORMATION. For age, 48; for comorbidity, average for age. My ER status—for estrogen receptor—was positive, that was good. Tumor grade was 2. On a 1 to 10 scale, I guessed. That's good, low side. Tumor size, 0.1 to 1.0 cm. Zero positive nodes. That was also good. My ten-year risk of relapse was 18 percent. Wait, that's almost a fifth. Four out of five people are alive without a recurrence of cancer in ten years. But one is not so lucky. Was I the one?

Ten years; that used to seem like a long time. At my ten-year college reunion everyone looked exactly the same except for the former homecoming queen, who had gained about a hundred pounds. Many of us were pleased with that detail, though I knew in my heart it was mean. The twenty-year college reunion was different. The women looked outstanding and the men not so good; they were bald and had bellies that hung out over their belts, and they still couldn't dance, though they acted as if in all that time no one had told them that simple truth. The men acted like they still were cute, you know, as Colin would say, "like they owned the place."

Oh, the women all looked great, because only the women who look outstanding go, Dana said. Not feeling quite Christie Brinkley? Stay home and send your regrets. Working out, doing yoga, had a recent touch-up of highlights? Then you could go.

At my twenty-five–year college reunion, I knew only a few people there. "Weren't you in marching band?" a woman asked me at the check-in table, who did not look at all familiar, not even if I squinted.

No, I was not. I was not in marching band. Nothing against marching band, but no.

Ten years. In ten years Colin grew from a toddler to a seventh grader; Weldon from a preschooler to a teenage driver; Brendan from being half my size to towering over me. I had spent ten years teaching at Northwestern; in that time having hundreds and hundreds of students in my classes. I wrote three books in ten years. It was ten years since I was divorced. I was alone for almost ten years and then I was in love. And then I was not.

You could do a lot in ten years. You could do a little. I would have to keep doing a lot.

On the right side was a graph in horizontal gray and black stripes. My chances of being alive in ten years? That was listed as 78.6 percent, with surgery only. That was a grade of C, not so good. With hormonal therapy, 88 percent chance. Better. With combined radiation and hormonal therapy, there was a 92 percent chance I would live to see Colin turn twenty-two. The paper said so. Nowhere on the paper did it say 100 percent. Nowhere.

My life was down to a printout, a thin sheet of paper I held in my hand, though the weight of it was a hundred million tons on my heart.

I knew it was possible that anyone could die at any time. I mean intellectually I knew this; we were not immortal. But most mornings before this all happened, when I made my bed, put the wet towels in the dryer, stirred the fruit in the yogurt, or pulled the car out of the driveway, it did not cross my mind all that much. I wanted to tell Dr. Rao about my Meg Ryan hair. Since the brachytherapy, my hair was thick and extracurly. It had this luscious messiness that was not its usual temperament. I woke up and it always looked fine.

"What do you mean?" Lisa asked.

"It's like my hair was blown dry from the inside out," I said.

Lisa wasn't buying my reasoning. No one had documented Meg Ryan hair as a side effect. "Are you using a different shampoo or conditioner?"

Dr. Rao gave me a prescription for tamoxifen and talked about how I would be taking it every day for the next five to ten years.

Tamoxifen. The name sounded like poison to me. It rhymed with *toxin.* And in a game of Scrabble, *toxin* would likely be the first derivative word that came to mind—every day for five years or more. I didn't know why I was so afraid of that small pill; perhaps it was because it held such power, because my survival depended on my taking it every day without fail.

I knew it blocked estrogen and that estrogen fed tumors. I understood it had been used for thirty years to treat breast cancer and that all the printed materials said the benefits outweighed the risks. But the side effects listed were not inconsequential: blood clots, stroke, uterine cancer, and cataracts. Oh, yes, and hot flashes, fatigue, headaches, nausea, vomiting, skin rash. Sounded like a pretty scary bucket list to me. Every day for five years. Then Dr. Rao said as an afterthought, yes, sometimes weight gain.

Wonderful. But I guess measure the weight gain against the recurrence, followed by dying and leaving your kids without a parent at home, and a little belly fat is fine. I could always wear jackets, to cover up the fat, I mean. Thank God tunics were in style.

I had a dream a few months later that I dropped the prescription plastic bottle of tamoxifen on the ground and a small white Maltese so tail-wagging sweet scooped down and licked up all the small pills. I was trying to grab the pills out of his mouth but couldn't get them before he swallowed all of them. Seconds later in my dream the dog collapsed and died. I woke up sweating and panicked.

"I recommend you have genetic testing on the tumor removed from your breast," Dr. Rao explained.

I nodded.

The test was the Oncotype DX breast cancer assessment, and it looked at twenty-one genes in the tumor tissue that could accurately determine the odds of recurrence by looking for specific biomarkers showing predisposition to other kinds of cancers. The test offered more information about the type of tumor it was and if I should have chemotherapy in addition to the radiation to significantly lower my chance of recurrence. They said recurrence, but what they meant is the chance you won't die by a certain time. A ten-year deadline. Or the chance that you will. The test, not covered by most insurance, came up with a recurrence score from 1 to 100, taking into account the biomarkers. I would wait two weeks for the results. I would later pay almost $4,000 for it. I had a list of questions for Dr. Rao, and she answered them, but it was as if she was speaking in slow motion; her words muffled and distorted through a screen of petroleum jelly. I just wanted to get out of her office, out of the building. I thanked her. I pretended that on the inside I was not hollowed out.

In the waiting room Mike was in the same chair. I handed him the piece of paper.

"Do you want me to talk to her?"

"No, let's go."

In the elevator I had to grip the handrails because I could not feel my legs and I started to cry. Mike held me up, his arm around my shoulder, gripping me. I thought I would faint; it felt like the closing moments of the Looney Tunes cartoons, when the circle of black tightens around Porky Pig and he stutters, "That's all, folks."

"She told me my chances of being alive in ten years," I said between sobs.

"But they are good," Mike said.

Mike was like my father, someone who was not prone to moods or ill temper; someone who would be the same kind soul on Tuesday as he was on the previous Thursday, and a thousand Thursdays to come. Like Johnny Carson was every night at 10:30, always in a good mood, always a smile on his face.

And here was Mike, taking a half day from the hospital for his sister-in-law. He was that same kind of man, to my sister of course, but really to all of us. He had always been good to my mother, like another son. He changed her light bulbs when she called, always available with medical advice and interventions. Talked to all her doctors, listened to her, invited her to dinner every Sunday night at their house; he cooked, mostly grilled fish like tilapia or salmon and vegetables. He was good to me and he was good to my boys. He came over to talk to the boys or go for a walk with their dog Haleigh, then Sammie. I was glad Mike was there.

When the elevator arrived at the main floor, we walked the criss-crossed hallways to the main lobby. My throat was parched; it felt as if all moisture in my body evaporated. I felt like my head was not connected to my body and I could fold to the floor like I was a paper doll.

"Let's sit," Mike said.

There by the deli counter with a clear case showing stacks of plastic containers of chef's salad, premade sandwiches, biscotti, coffee, and juice, I cried. Nurses and doctors and visitors were buying lunch and snacks and going about their day because no one had just told them their chances of being alive in ten years. I couldn't hold it in. I cried. The wet bursts were hiccupping hard because my boys weren't there and I knew I couldn't cry like this at home. I cried in front of twenty people eating a late lunch because I had to be a vision of strength and a comfort to the boys at home later. My surgery and radiation scared them. I learned that teenage boys who have been abandoned by a parent don't take well to the illness of the only parent they have left to care for them. They became aggressive, irritable, caustic to me and to each other.

"I didn't expect them to be mean," I told Susy when she brought over dinner for all of us.

"Oh, those wonderful boys. They are so scared," she said.

I knew she was right. I knew it was scary for them. But for some reason I thought that fear would manifest itself as them trying to take care of me, being very low maintenance, taking care of themselves, not requiring more of me, certainly not fighting with each other and definitely not talking back to me. I pictured them being sweet and solicitous, perhaps throwing in an extra load of laundry. What the heck, making me a cup of tea. I don't know what in the hell I was thinking.

While Weldon held it together better than the other two, I would say my cancer made them mad as hell. And they were mad as hell at me. I was the one who was sick; how dare I do this? You could see it in their eyes, the skittishness, the doubt; they were pissed off. When they would ask how I was, they would leave the room before my answer; they would not want to know any details. I had to be OK. Brendan could be sweet, you could see him trying, when he made me breakfast or when he bought me hand cream, trying so hard to be caring, when I could see how scared he was.

What's next? Will you die next?

Colin had a harder time and was uncharacteristically argumentative with me and with his brothers. One night Colin would not stop arguing with me, so I called Madeleine for help; she sent Mike over to get Colin for a few hours. Absorbing their fears and their anger was exhausting. I would lie down on the couch for a half hour and sleep for five hours.

"I've never seen you take a nap," Colin said.

I was so tired; a bone-deep weariness I couldn't shake or emerge from immediately. After surgery, even after the abbreviated radiation treatments, for about a month, I woke up tired. I started out feeling like it was the end of the day. My head felt swollen, I couldn't think clearly, I couldn't take care of everyone else while they were screaming for me to do more please so they didn't feel afraid. But I kept going.

The night after my third day of radiation was parent-teacher conferences at the high school. I met with six of Weldon's teachers. The next night I would meet with six of Brendan's, second floor, fourth floor, third floor, second floor, all right after radiation. Most of the conferences were six minutes apart; some sessions had breaks in between. In the four-floor high school, many of the sessions were two floors apart. First was room 411 with Mr. Goldberg for history, down to 217 for math, back up to 417 for Spanish, down to 333. I sat in the third-floor hallway outside the classroom waiting for my time with Weldon's English teacher, Brendan Lee, Weldon's favorite. My conference was from 6:42 to 6:48. I would talk fast. I had a few minutes to get to room 361 for Mr. Potts. Then down to 284 for Mr. Martinek, science.

"What's wrong with you? What makes you look so tired?" asked another woman I had known since our oldest children were in preschool together. She wasn't a good friend. It was different out in the noncancer world. Questions were curt. Judgments were made.

"Must be the radiation after the surgery," I answered and went back to the pile of papers in my lap from the other teachers, on top of the legal pad where I had taken notes on comments about Weldon and Brendan.

"Oh, sorry. I didn't know." And she didn't ask me any questions.

My work life went on. Wrestling went on, basketball for Colin, dinners in the room off the kitchen, loads of whites and loads of colors separated every morning. Gas in the car. Checks to pay the bills, boots and sneakers piled in the mudroom needing to be straightened. Dishwasher to load and unload, kitchen floor to sweep. Homework to proofread, forms to sign.

A few weeks later I sat in the stands watching one of Colin's games talking with Alex's mom, who was an emergency room doctor.

"The tamoxifen upsets my stomach," I told her.

"Eat jelly beans. One at a time. Licorice ones will help. The pectin and the sugar will soothe your stomach. Try it," Sherry said. "Get the cheap ones; for some reason they work better."

So I sat in the stands and in meetings with brightly colored jelly beans in my pocket. It was a small solution, one bite at a time.

Part Three

REVERSAL

13

STANDS

December 2006–January 2007

The day before Christmas Eve there was a local tournament for Weldon, then the day before New Year's Eve a tournament in Elmwood, Ohio. I couldn't get away for that one; I stayed home with Colin and Brendan. Weldon went with the team. Then four more wrestling tournaments were at local high schools, followed by the Huskie tournament at home in the field house. Weldon won that 140-pound championship with a pin. That pin and others from the team pushed Oak Park to win the invitational tournament with 263 points.

The following Friday night was a dual meet at another local high school, Lyons Township. The boys' father had left a message on the house answering machine a few days earlier that he was in town from Amsterdam. Surprise. He had not spoken to the boys in two months. I listened to it, told the boys he called, and no one called him back. Weldon said his father had also left him a message on his cell. I had not spoken to his father, but I knew he must be watching Weldon's wrestling record online for the season.

"Dad e-mailed me about my match," Weldon said. "He said he wanted to see me wrestle." Then he added, "I blocked his e-mail address."

Weldon was annoyed at my questions for more details.

"I don't want him there; he is not going to ruin this for me. I can't be distracted," he said.

I didn't know what it would be like being monitored online by a phantom father, but I imagined it was something like a version of a scene I saw in the 1937 movie *Stella Dallas*, starring Barbara Stanwyck. I loved the old black-and-white movies that were romantic and emotional with grandly feminine characters in bias-cut satin dresses swooning over handsome men with mustaches. At the end of the movie, Stella watched her daughter Laurel's wedding from outside the window of the house her ex-husband shared with his new wife.

I knew their father would go to the meet; he loved being in control of a surprise, even if no one wanted it. Both Brendan and Weldon went on the team bus to Lyons. Colin went to a friend's house. I took my place in the stands with the other Huskie parents and told Paula, Kake, and Caryn that I was nervous. They sat closer to me.

I saw him immediately. Their father was standing on the top stair in one corner of the gym, wearing a bright red sweater, with both his arms stretched out holding onto the wall. You could not miss him. Anyone glancing up at the stands from anywhere would see him, a half-body length above the crowd, the only one in bright red and the only one with outstretched arms.

"He's looking right at you," Nancy said.

I watched Brendan's junior varsity match and waited for the 140 varsity match, wondering if Weldon noticed his dad. Weldon paced back and forth before his match as he usually did, and jumped high in place bending his knees beneath him in this limber frog move that had become his trademark. I watched his face, more stern than usual. He jumped about four feet in the air from a standing position, his legs tucked tightly under him. Over and over.

Weldon was pushing really hard, and there was something about his mood, something about the way he wrestled, so driven, so intense.

He knew he was being watched. He won 20–5, another technical. Brendan was sitting in the stands on the opposite side of the gym from the spectators, with his junior varsity teammates. I watched him to see if he noticed his father and if Brendan would go to speak to him. After Weldon wrestled, I glanced over at the top deck in the stands where his father had been standing. He was gone. I went down to the floor to speak to Weldon after his win.

"Are you OK?" I asked.

Sweat was pouring down his face and he was clearly agitated.

"He better not be in the parking lot," he said.

"No, he's gone," I said.

Then I walked over to the stands and asked Brendan, "Did you see your dad?"

"No, was he here?"

When the dual was over, I went to the parking lot, looking behind me, around me, nervous that he would pop up out of the shadows. But he had disappeared.

We were less than a month away from the 2007 state championships. In July 2006 I had made hotel reservations online for the upcoming February Illinois High School Association (IHSA) Individual championships. The year before when Weldon made it to state, I was unprepared, panicked, and couldn't get a room when he won regionals. All nearby hotel rooms were booked. Not ever having had this experience, I had no idea that parents of wrestlers booked a year in advance, confident they would need to attend because their sons would have winning seasons that qualified them for state.

So I went online the year before just days before state and called every hotel and motel in a ten-mile radius with no luck. I knew I couldn't drive the three hours each way there and back safely in one day. When I told him about not having a room, the boys' uncle Mark somehow managed to book a room for Colin, Brendan, and me at the local Holiday Inn. Mark then drove down to meet us and watched Weldon.

I knew Weldon would qualify for state again. I was more convinced of it every time he wrestled. We were less than a month away from the finals and he was winning almost every match. Reserving the room six months ahead of time was easy; now all he needed to do was keep winning. A lot of us Huskies parents had our eyes set on state for the boys.

A few days after he appeared in the stands at Lyons, the boys' dad left a voice mail on Weldon's cell. "I have tickets for state and a hotel room . . ." Weldon hung up and screamed for me; I was upstairs in my room.

"Mom!" Weldon bounded up the front stairs two or three at a time. "Mom! Tell him not to come. Tell him I don't want him there." Weldon was extremely upset, pacing, shouting. "He said he has tickets and a room!"

I felt like a mother lion protecting her cub from a python that had slithered in from the nearby grass.

"OK, I will, OK," I said.

I called his father's cell phone. He answered. I didn't know if he was local or back in the Netherlands. I started shouting. "Leave Weldon alone right now. Do not ruin this for him. Do not come to state. Do not take this away from him."

"Let me explain," he said.

"No more explanations, no more. You will not hurt him anymore. I will not let you." Now I was frantic. "He told you what he wants. You must respect him. Don't come."

"Relax," he said.

I couldn't. The other two boys came upstairs to see what was wrong.

"I mean it. You cannot ruin this for Weldon. You have done enough. I will not let you."

I hung up and called his mother. I told her that she needed to tell her son to respect Weldon's wishes. She said she would. Five minutes later she called me back.

"Dear, he said he has no plans to go. He said he left a message for Weldon that he had tickets for state and he could give them to any friends of his who needed them or any families who wanted the room."

I felt stupid. "Thank you," I said.

I hung up and told Weldon what his grandmother said.

"Did you listen to the whole message?" I asked Weldon.

"No."

"Let me listen."

The full message was just as his mother said. I laughed out loud. All that roaring for nothing. I took a deep breath and called his father back. "No, thank you, no one needs the tickets. I should not have yelled, but Weldon told me I needed to tell you not to come."

14

GESTURE

February 16–17, 2007

pulled to the curb outside Dorothea's apartment at 6 in the morning on Friday. It was still dark and bitterly cold, four below zero, the kind of dagger-sharp chill that hurt your nostrils when you breathed and made you feel as if your clothes were made of cellophane. Snowflakes fell like promises. Brendan and Colin were stretched in the middle and third seats, each with a pillow and blanket, ready to doze on the 126-mile drive to see their older brother compete in the individual state finals. I'd called the younger two boys out of school the night before; Weldon had gone with the team on the bus Thursday night.

It was Weldon's second year at the IHSA Individual State Wrestling Tournament, but as a senior, this was his last chance to make it to the finals stand, the winner's boxes. Dorothea's son, Dan, was wrestling as a sophomore at 145 pounds, one weight class above Weldon's.

I'd gotten up by 5 AM, making sure I had everyone's overnight bags by the door. I packed sandwiches, fruit, snacks, soda, water, and

Gatorade for the day. The year before when Weldon competed at state, I'd learned that pretty much all the concession stands inside the arena offered was fried, refried, batter dipped, cheese or chocolate-smothered, and prohibitively expensive. Enormous scoops of ice cream in waffle cones, four-dollar fountain drinks, huge wedges of pie with fistfuls of vanilla ice cream on top, soft pretzels the size of catchers' mitts. You could spend twenty dollars on lunch, easy. I also knew we would have to hide the food we brought from home in our coat pockets, as you were not allowed to take any coolers or food into the arena. They checked purses and bags. Dorothea ended up stowing some oranges in her sweater. We figured no one was going to frisk her.

We had a large entourage of parents from Oak Park and River Forest High School that year—nine wrestlers plus Coach Powell and all the varsity, freshmen, junior varsity, and youth wrestling coaches too. The youth coach took a group of Little Huskies in a van to watch. Every one of the boys on our team, and every team from across the state, Class A and Class AA (this was two years before Class AAA was added), were aiming for first place ideally, but a medal for second, third, or fourth would be great. Other members of the Huskies team had painted a sign for the Oak Park High School student center with the names of state-bound wrestlers and their weights alongside an outline of the state of Illinois. "Good luck at State!" it read in the center. Painted in blue were the names and records of the eight Huskies wrestlers headed to state—a huge number from the roster.

I booked a room at the local Ramada. We would drive back Saturday night, no matter how late. I was hoping it would be late and that Weldon would be the champion; there was chatter at the high school that he could win it all. His math teacher gave everyone in Weldon's class extra-credit points because he made it to state. I didn't teach on Fridays and brought my laptop so I could catch up on work, grade papers, or respond to e-mails when I could, in between wrestling matches high up in the stands. Twenty-four of us were seated in Section B for Friday and Saturday.

The boys slept most of the way there; Dorothea and I talked about our sons, our lives, and our work. We had to park about a block away in the lots surrounding the arena; it felt appreciably colder and windier, the temperature on a local sign read –9 degrees. A line of more than one hundred parka and fleece–clad parents and teens stretched down the snaking walkway to the glass-enclosed ticket booth to buy tickets, all of them hopping in place or rubbing their hands and face to try to stay warm. I apologetically rushed past them into the booth to the will-call window and picked up the block of tickets with my name on it.

From the outside, the University of Illinois Assembly Hall looked like an enormous white, glass, and metal spaceship that seemed to have landed amid the cornfields, low campus buildings, and flat, empty stretches of lawn and asphalt surrounding it on campus. What had been green in the summer and fall was now snow and ice–covered. Inside, the hall itself dwarfed the swirling dance of athletes, coaches, and parents. The arena held sixteen thousand people, and it was nearly filled to capacity, just as it had been years earlier for the Rolling Stones, U2, and Tina Turner. The throbbing anticipation was palpable.

I imagined that as a wrestler on the floor of the arena, with six mats of contrasting orange and blue circles, standing at the center of your mat, you would feel like a rock star: the cheering crowds, the wish that you would be the one with your arm raised in victory. For every athlete who made it this far, it was a long way from early Sunday mornings of youth wrestling in the high school gyms.

Some of the young men on the floor of the arena looked moonlight pale, their faces gaunt, their bodies tightly muscular. They all carried themselves with confidence, having earned their place to compete after beating as many as forty other wrestlers along the way during the season, all of whom dreamed of coming here and standing inside the arena wearing his team's singlet, his coach sitting at the edge of the mat calculating every move.

"Some of the other teams with their neat warmup suits and trimmed hair look like boy bands," Caryn said.

Even though the wrestlers on our team had matching team shirts and warmups, they tended not to wear them to tournaments.

"Our boys look like wrestlers," she said.

A group of four couples in their late sixties were seated in the row in front of us, carefully marking each winner in every weight class on their programs. After a few hours of observing them engrossed in certain contests and chatting about all the wrestlers, I asked, "So do you have a grandson or relative wrestling today?"

"Oh, no," one of the men responded. "We do this for fun."

Weldon had a bye the first round, meaning he was excused from wrestling in the preliminaries. Every first-place winner of every sectional had a bye when he advanced to the state finals. The top three sectional placers made it to state, and the second and third placers at regionals faced each other in the preliminary round.

Weldon faced a wrestler from Plainfield with a season record of 37 wins and 3 losses; slightly better than Weldon's, at 32–4. Weldon had wrestled him at state in 2006, and lost to him 9–3. I moved from my seat in the stands to the railings to watch Weldon face him on the mat, as did Colin and Brendan. We were screaming for him; Colin was shooting video. Weldon got back points and took his opponent down, but he cut him twice, earning his opponent two points.

It was the only time you could stand by the railing; otherwise the security guards and ushers politely but firmly told you to get back to your seat. You hoped the opponent's parent was nowhere near you, because the last thing you needed to hear up close was some other parent urging at the top of his lungs for his son to annihilate yours. This is where wrestlers ended up if they dared to be great. This was the goal. This was the bonus of working so hard.

Weldon lost the match 6–5, close; the last few seconds felt as if they passed in slow motion. The striped-shirted ref raised the other wrestler's hand in the air and I wanted to cry.

It was good enough just to be here, I practiced telling him, *you got this far, it was fine, it was all right, it was enough. Be proud.*

When the match was over, Weldon crossed over the mat to shake the hand of the Plainfield coach, went back to speak to Powell, and both of them headed to the sidelines. I expected Powell to put his hand on Weldon's shoulder, console him, pat him on the back. But Powell was screaming at him, animatedly gesturing, his arms moving wildly, like I had never seen him do before to any wrestler, let alone Weldon, whose head was hung, nodding. Powell must have yelled at him for a full five or six minutes.

The boys and I walked back to our seats in the stands, the other parents offering their kind words. Paula gave me a hug. It was my instinct to want to hug Weldon, but he was down in the team section with the competing wrestlers and coaches, Powell still giving it to him pretty good. I was angry Powell yelled at him.

The last thing he needed was Powell berating him. Of course Weldon knew he let him down, of course he felt bad. Why make it worse?

According to Weldon, it was exactly what he needed.

"Powell yelled at me because I blew it. He wanted me to go to the finals," Weldon explained later. "I didn't have the belief or the confidence. Nothing happens miraculously unless you make it happen. I didn't wrestle to win," Weldon said. He said Powell told him, "Don't stop now. Let's get third."

Hours passed; individual dramas played out over and over again on each mat for each wrestler, some elated to win, their parents jumping and screaming and hugging each other; some acting like gorillas flexing and puffing up their chests, taunting the opposing coach after a win. Still some other wrestlers cried, nearly inconsolable if they lost, shoulders shaking as they walked off the mat, sobbing into the sweatpants they picked up from the floor where they had dropped them. All of it happening at once, on four mats of wrestling for Class AA teams, two mats for Class A teams.

Some boys sat restless in the stands with their teams, humpbacks of ice bags taped to their shoulders or backs, staring straight ahead as they waited. All of it was as loud as the middle of a construction site with drills piercing cement, all of it confusing. Six matches were ongoing at all times relentlessly, with everyone moving—up and down in the stands, back and forth to the concessions. A constant flow of fans and athletes, back and forth, whistles blowing incessantly on the mats, winners every few minutes, losers just as often. Outside it was still bitterly cold and snowing.

"Did you ever think you would watch five hundred wrestling matches in one day?" asked Tom, a father of three sons, two of whom were wrestlers on our team. That is how many they had per day and more.

Weldon would have a chance at the wrestle-backs on Saturday. That was a part of wrestling I loved. You lost once, but your loss did not define you. You could come back up to the championship through wrestle-backs, the consolation round. If the person who beat you kept winning and made it to the quarterfinal matches, you were eligible to compete in the consolation bracket; you were still in.

All of us from the Oak Park wrestling family made plans for dinner together. I called around town for reservations, but no restaurant could take our crowd of about twenty-four. Not the local Olive Garden or the hamburger and pizza spots, not even the Jolly Roger where about thirty of us had eaten the year earlier. It was a 1960s time warp of a restaurant that served retro food like shrimp cocktail, cottage cheese with French dressing, and large pizzas to feed ten that cost the same as a single sandwich from Panera. But this year it was closed. We gave up trying to find a spot and agreed to meet back in the lobby of our motel, where we ordered about ten pizzas and ate every morsel of them.

Weldon called me from one of the team's hotel rooms.

"Did you get a chance to rinse out your singlet in the sink?" I asked. He was sharing a room with about six other wrestlers.

"No," he said, as if that was the dumbest thing he ever heard.

Saturday weigh-ins were at 6 AM for the athletes, plus skin checks. No wrestler can have a rash—MRSA, impetigo, ringworm, anything suspicious or contagious. Paul was planning to drive down and be at the arena by 9 AM, but it was snowing hard in Chicago and on the way to Champaign visibility was near zero; several inches of snow were expected. Paul called to say I-57 was closed because cars were wiping out on the ice. He decided to turn back to go home.

Weldon won his first match of the morning 6–4. It didn't look easy for him, but Weldon appeared much more confident, a different wrestler than the night before. Later that morning, Weldon competed against a senior from Conant High School with a record of 32–10. Weldon beat him 13–4, a huge win, and he almost pinned him. I was screaming and clapping and cheering so much my throat was hoarse. Brendan and Colin were ecstatic.

In the next match Weldon was up against a West Aurora wrestler who had a season record of 36–4. If Weldon won this match, he would be a placer at state. He could win third, fourth, or fifth. He could get a medal. The boys and I, plus several of the team parents, went to the railing to get as close as we could. I was wearing my Huskies Wrestling Family T-shirt, as were Colin and Brendan.

Weldon took his opponent down, again, and again. Three times. And in the last period, he won 7–2. Colin was jumping up and down and we were all hugging each other, the arena spotlight on Weldon, thousands of people cheering.

The ref held Weldon's hand in the air, and he stood straight, with a look that he was full of the moment and of himself. With his one arm raised, Weldon turned to where I was in the stands. With his free hand, he pointed directly to me and held it there for what was only a few seconds but felt like hours.

I gasped, held my hand in front of my mouth, and started to cry. He walked off the mat and leapt into Coach Powell's arms. I went back to my seat and felt a buffet of emotions, from relief, joy, pride, and gratitude to elation.

Look what my son could do. See who he is.

"It's OK, Mom," Colin said, I guess embarrassed by my sobbing.

"I love you, Mom," Brendan said as he hugged me.

It reminded me of when Colin was in kindergarten during the Valentine's Day event called "Big Hearts, Little Hands." Bill's wife, Madonna, had created the school's annual tradition of the afternoon musical recital for families and the local senior community, followed by a formal tea in the gymnasium. The little girls wore their pink-and-red party dresses and the boys wore suits and clip-on ties, stiff-collared shirts tucked hastily into neatly pressed pants. The children sang a few songs, including the 1962 Woody Guthrie song, "I'm Gonna Mail Myself to You."

For the recital and tea, I picked up my mother at her house, pushed her wheelchair to the end of the row in the school auditorium, and we watched as the rows of boys and girls squirmed and jiggled through the lyrics. They sang, "I'm gonna wrap myself in paper, I'm gonna daub myself with glue, Stick some stamps on top of my head; I'm gonna mail myself to you." On the last line, every other student in the stands arranged on the stage pointed to Mrs. Halter, the music teacher in the orchestra pit. Not Colin. After weeks of practice and finally having every one of the thirty or so students pointing to her on cue, Colin turned to his right and pointed to me. My mother and I laughed.

"Why would I want to mail myself to the music teacher?" Colin said when I asked him about it later.

After Weldon's win, Brendan, Colin, and I went to the concessions stands. I felt so giddy I bought three overpriced gray hooded sweatshirts for the boys, with the official IHSA Individual Wrestling State Championship logo on the front. I signed up for the official photos to be mailed to me. I ordered the plaque. Heck, I would have ordered a pony if they sold one. On the sweatshirt for Weldon, I had the saleswoman iron on letters on the back that read his name, plus 140 ALL STATE. For Brendan, I had her iron on his name, plus THE NEXT ONE. For Colin, I asked her to iron on his last name, plus III. The two boys put on the sweatshirts immediately and we held onto Weldon's to give to him later. He would get what he came for; he would stand with the champions on the winner's boxes.

Hours later Weldon wrestled a Geneseo wrestler with a 28–1 record. Weldon won 3–2, a tough, pretty even match. He could win third or fourth now. At the end of the match, Weldon knew he was a placer. He was slated next to wrestle a Glenbard North wrestler with a 33–5 record for the season, one more win than Weldon but also one more loss. We went down to the railing and screamed for him, but Weldon couldn't seem to score on him. His opponent was several inches shorter than Weldon, a way different build, not lanky and muscular, more compact. Weldon lost 6–1, earning him fourth place. This was good enough and I knew Weldon was pleased. When he walked away from the mat, I knew he still felt proud.

When the 140 championship was over, a ceremony was held on the main floor, as it was for every championship of every weight class. Only one parent was allowed to take photos near the winner's boxes, where all the boys stood after the red, white, and blue ribboned gold medals were placed on their necks. I reported to Aisle A26 and stood next to the fathers or mothers of the top three winners. In some of the photographs Weldon's face was marked with bruises and cuts, the medal around his neck hanging to the middle of his blue-and-orange Oak Park wrestling sweatshirt. In other shots, he was smiling, but he looked tired, spent, young.

After watching Peter, our team's heavyweight, take second place, Dorothea and I raced to the car in the iced night cold, the snow glistening in the parking lot like spun sugar, Brendan and Colin tired and eager to sleep. We drove the three hours home in a caravan, three families in a row following each other on the unlit stretch of highway. Weldon rode in the van with the team. He said on the way home all the wrestlers stopped at McDonald's and he ate four cheeseburgers. He wouldn't have to weigh 140 pounds for a very long time, if ever.

When we got home, our next-door neighbors, who had been following Weldon's wins online, put a sign on our front door and draped toilet paper on the small evergreens that flanked the entrance, a tradition in the suburb where we lived when someone won at state in any sport.

A few days later, Powell e-mailed the Huskie Wrestling Family:

The wrestling coaches often ask our wrestlers to do things that parents, friends, teachers, and even the wrestlers themselves have difficulty under-standing. We ask our athletes to wrestle with the following questions: "If you work the hardest and the smartest, do you get the most? Is it OK to be fanatical about something; giving up the balance in life so many people believe is important?" The answer from five Huskie wrestlers would be yes. Ellis, Lillashawn, Weldon, Peter L., and Peter K. all made it to the second day of the Individual State Wrestling tournament in Champaign this weekend. Under grueling conditions, each of these young men wrestled with the passion and heart that only a person who has really sacrificed could. Preparations for the 2007 State Tournament were exhausting. To truly document all of the work these young men have done would take thousands of pages. They have given up so much. They have endured pain and anguish beyond what most people reading this could comprehend. They have trained 365 days in each of the last several years. Forgoing many typical teenage experiences and choosing to mentally and physically suffer, to reach goals promised by coaches, takes unbelievable character and faith. As big win after big win rolled in this weekend, the answers to the above questions became clear.

Coach Powell then offered a synopsis of each wrestler's highlights. For Weldon he wrote:

Weldon will graduate the school as the most entertaining, most dynamic wrestler ever. It is at times hard to tell whether one is watching a wrestling match or a dance performance. With speed, grace and agility, all developed through relentless work, Weldon has crushed the previous takedown record at the school on his way to the All-State stand this past weekend. Weldon defeated two nationally ranked opponents this weekend. He has already told me the answer—it was worth it. The Team places sixth in the standings this weekend. This is the best finish in School History! These five wrestlers contributed. With different physical assets and five completely different styles, each of these young men has the most important things in common. They have worked the hardest and the smartest. They have sacrificed the most to discover potential that they did not previously know they had. We are very proud of the young men and their teammates who every day live a lifestyle unfathomable by most.

In relentless pursuit,
Michael Powell

"Nothing is as satisfying as having your hand raised," Weldon told me later. "I can't describe it. It's recognition and happiness, contentment. If you train that hard, you're supposed to win. When you lose you have to think about why you lost and what you're going to do to get better. Fourth isn't bad; it could have been better. Of course it was worth it."

The outdoor marquee at the high school soccer fields ran the names of the boys who placed at state flashing in neon. Paula drove by and took photos. I put a photo of Weldon on my bulletin board outside my office at work. The next week were team state finals, anticlimactic after the individual competition.

A few weeks later at the wrestling banquet in the school's north cafeteria, every wrestler and his family from freshman to varsity brought a dish for the potluck collection of comfort food that ranged from chicken wings and fried chicken to lasagna and salad, desserts and cookies. Weeks after the season ended and making weight was over, the boys all looked rounder, their cheekbones no longer as prominent, their faces full, their hair growing back from the clean-shaven bald they all sported in December.

When he called each wrestler to the podium, Powell talked about him with keen detail, respect, and personal insight—telling jokes, complimenting him, showing how well he knew each wrestler. Most years, when he talked about the seniors, he fought back tears.

"We try to give the boys the most difficult, trying, comprehensive, loving, athletic experience you can have. When you love someone enough, you can have high expectations," Powell said. "You can have great athletes and they can find out what it means to be men."

That afternoon Weldon won the MVP (most valuable player) award along with Peter Kowalczuk. Weldon was listed in the program for making it to US Nationals off-season for Team Illinois, as well as Junior Nationals and as an Academic All-Conference wrestler. He was All-Conference as well. His season record was 37–6, making it to the "Thirty Wins a Season" list with five other teammates. He won the Takedown King award, for 223 takedowns that season, a record for the school that was not broken until two years later.

Powell called Weldon to the podium. Weldon stood beside him, hands clasped in front of him.

"He was such a terrible wrestler his freshman year," Powell said. Everyone laughed.

And then he talked about what kind of man he was now. "I would want my daughter to marry him," Powell said. "I want him for a son."

15

BANKRUPT

July 2, 2007

Thankfully, bankruptcy court was different than divorce court, more like traffic court or the waiting area of the Department of Motor Vehicles. Luckily, no one was taking a photo of me that day that I had to carry around in my wallet for four years.

Still I wanted to look responsible, respectable; I wanted to show the trustee that I was not at fault, I was not delinquent. My former husband had filed for Chapter 7, claiming he had no assets to pay any of his debts, including child support. It was three years after he moved away, two years after he stopped paying child support, and almost one year after he last saw his three sons. I was his biggest creditor; really, the boys were. The lump sum of unpaid child support at that time was approaching six figures, more if you added the refused extraordinary medical expenses he was ordered to pay in the original divorce decree. And tens of thousands every year when you added in college expenses.

It was an amount that was growing and eventually would reach more than $300,000.

"I choose not to participate in Brendan's braces at this time," their dad told me two years earlier when I informed him of his court-ordered share of the bill.

The collectors on his defaulted law school loans had been calling our house for about three years, asking for him, insisting he lived there over my denials. My byline is my maiden name and I did not change my name to his when I got married, as I had a decade-long journalism reputation under that byline by then.

Sometimes the boys said their father was dead when the collection agency asked to speak to him on the phone. I was never listed on any law school loan paperwork as responsible for it, even though we were married at the time that he borrowed. Our current home was never an address where he lived; I moved there with the boys a year after the divorce. But the collectors hounded me, they hounded us. Letters, phone calls.

Even when I explained to the collectors that he likely owed me more than he owed them, they were not understanding or even civil and kept calling the house and demanding to speak to him. Early in the morning, late at night, on weekends. If we were all home and I could account for each of the boys, we stopped picking up any call at home that was an 800 number or listed as "private number" on caller ID. It was either the law loans people or the solicitors for aluminum siding. We had a brick house.

A few weeks before on my forty-ninth birthday, June 5, a summons of this meeting of creditors arrived at our house. The notice said it would be held in the office of Allan DeMars, a partner in the Chicago firm of Spiegel & DeMars. I was sure the timing of the delivery was deliberate. My former husband had e-mailed me the same day with an e-birthday card saying I didn't look fifty. Never mind he had not seen me in two years. Never mind I was one year shy of fifty anyway; it's those kinds of details he often forgot. A few weeks later I received a polite letter from DeMars informing me of my rights as a creditor and the process of collecting back child support. The trustee and the state of Illinois would be able to help.

The hearing was not about me, it was about their dad; really, it was about the boys and what I needed to do for them. I placed in my briefcase files and letters plus an eight-by-ten framed color photo of the boys taken in Michigan, laughing. I thought if the hearing steered away from my purpose of collecting child support, I would place the photo of the boys on the desk and remind their dad exactly who it was he had stopped supporting. Look at them. They are of you. OK, it was a little *Judge Judy*, but so what.

Around my neck I wore my father's gold medal of the Blessed Virgin Mary. It weighed heavy on my chest, underneath the simple black top. I guess I was hoping it brought me peace of mind and luck, reminded me of saying the Rosary every night after dinner while I was growing up. Wearing his medal made me feel close to my dad; he was a good father who died in 1988 before any of my sons were born. Seeing me go through this now would have made my father cry, and it would have also made him hell-furious.

I drove downtown, parked, and walked to my sister's firm where I met with her law partner, Bob, my attorney. We walked the block south to court. We showed our driver's licenses, registered, and were given bar-coded green-and-white stickers that would allow us into the hearing. When we got to the thirty-third floor, my ex-husband was there sitting near the door of room 3360. The sight of him made my stomach cartwheel.

My former husband was wearing tawny crushed velvet pants and a silky yellow shirt—an absurd outfit that made him look like Rod Stewart or an *American Idol* contestant voted off early in the season, and too silly for a bankruptcy hearing. He was more slender than I remembered, his brown hair rock-star long. He was remarkably tan, his skin the burnished tortoise color of someone who sunbathed for a living. That must be what he did with his time and why he claimed he only made $300 that year.

I headed to the right of the room with Bob. Dozens of sad people appeared consumed by a similar pathos, the same deflated admission that life was hard, money was elusive, and this was a destination of last resort. No one looked pleased to be there.

Most everyone in the waiting area looked down at their shoes and avoided eye contact.

We sat a few rows in front of my former husband, with our backs to him. Pink sheets of paper laminated in plastic pinned to cork bulletin boards reminded everyone to have their driver's license and proof of social security number ready. The debtors needed to prove who they were.

Thirty minutes later, his name was called.

The trustee's office was the size of our breakfast room at home or a small office. Molded blue plastic and chrome chairs, plain walls, Formica desk. The trustee looked like a car salesman: white hair, oblong face, wire-rimmed glasses, plain white shirt, tie, no jacket. It was fitting as his office resembled one of the small offices in a car showroom where they insisted you could not get any more off the list price and you were lucky to get this car because someone else wanted it today. Allan DeMars was polite and straightforward. *He must have heard some doozies*, I thought. This was a man who couldn't be shocked.

He introduced the federal US bankruptcy trustee seated in the back row of the room. I sat two seats away from the boys' father, with Bob seated between us, across from the trustee's neat desk. After asking permission, DeMars turned on a small black tape recorder, one that looked like something Radio Shack sold in the 1980s, not digital but with real tape. I wonder if it worked.

He swore in my ex-husband under oath. DeMars asked him his name. He asked him his address. My former husband gave the address of his elderly parents as his own, a place he stayed when he was in the United States no more than thirty days a year.

"I object," I said with a loud, broad indignation, having seen more than a few *Boston Legal* episodes. I felt like the Candice Bergen character, without the facelift.

"You can't object," DeMars said politely. "He is under oath and subject to perjury. You will have time to question him later," he explained.

I fidgeted and my heart raced.

"Relax," Bob whispered.

But it was all coming back. The deceit, the 10 percent truths sold as reality, the arrogance. Perhaps less than ten minutes later, the trustee was finished.

"Do you have any questions?" he asked me.

"Yes, and I need about twenty minutes," I said, and pulled out my file from my briefcase.

"All you have is five," DeMars responded matter-of-factly.

He asked my ex-husband if he would submit voluntarily to questioning by his creditor.

My former husband mumbled something.

"You can be subpoenaed to answer questions at another time and place, but it is easier to do it now, right here," DeMars said. "As your creditor, she has the legal right to ask you any questions pertaining to assets."

He agreed.

"Where do you live more than three hundred days a year?" I asked him, my voice shaking.

He placed his hand over his mouth and gave his address in the Netherlands.

"Do you have an Illinois driver's license?"

He said he did.

"How can that be if you are not an Illinois resident?"

He didn't answer.

"Keep your questions to the subject of assets," DeMars said, shuffling papers on his desk.

"How could you afford the $1,600 airfare from Amsterdam to Chicago three times this year if you have no money?" I asked.

"My ex-wife paid for one trip," he responded without looking up.

"Your second ex-wife," I reminded him.

He said Ingrid, his current partner, paid for the other two trips.

"How can you afford to have counsel from Skadden, Arps, Slate, Meagher & Flom?" I asked. It is a prestigious top-shelf law firm.

"My attorney is my cousin," he said clearly annoyed.

"And he's Brendan's godfather," I snapped.

"Your questions must be limited to the topic of assets," the trustee said again. "Please have your client ask questions pertaining only to assets," he said to Bob.

But I had other questions.

"How could it be possible without assets to afford the $11,000 annual tuition to Wisdom University?"

This was my long shot. I inquired about the school that was an offshoot of Damanhur, the spiritual organization he told me he had belonged to for more than five years. He had told me years earlier he was earning a degree to become a spiritual healer at the University of Turin in Italy. I told him on many occasions that he was better off banking on his law degree from a top midwestern law school to land a job.

God bless Google. The night before the hearing I went hunting for more information on him on the Internet. I figured that since he could not speak Italian, he wasn't really studying at the University of Turin, since the site was in Italian and it appeared all course work was in Italian. So I typed in "spiritual university in Turin and Damanhur." I had surmised that he attended a university in Turin run by Damanhur, the spiritual community described on its website as "a Federation of communities with over 800 citizens, a social and political structure, a Constitution, economic activities, its own currency, schools and a daily paper."

No wonder he didn't pay child support; his cult has its own currency.

Months earlier I found his website for Damanhur consultations by typing in his name. Both he and Ingrid were pictured in the same deep red color shirt; she was smiling brilliantly and he looked uncomfortable, as if he had been caught in a lie.

Their site explained they offered spiritual trips to Egypt and Italy, and the costs. "Let a Wonder of the Ancient World, The Alhambra in Granada, Spain Inspire You" read the brochure in .pdf form with his name listed as coach and his home address in Delft. The website was in Dutch, but I clicked for an English translation.

His bio read:

I turn the tales and the history of the Alhambra into reality for you. These myths and legends are key to an inspiring world full of wonders and mystery. Using my qualities as an American lawyer, journalist and philosopher, I will bring these strange places to your life.

With the prices listed for these trips, clearly he would make more than $300 a year.

The text continued, "It also has a university that attracts philosophical and spiritual students from all over the world. Damanhur is named after an Egyptian city located one hundred miles northwest of Cairo in the middle of the western Delta," the website stated. "It was once the site of the city of Tmn-Hor, dedicated to the god Horus."

The text went on. "Damanhur exists to build and service its Temple of Humankind which the community has been building deep within a mountain for nearly two decades."

Areas of study include Dancing with the Missionary, Environmental Intimacy, and Intermediate Digital and Ancient Storytelling. I printed out twenty-four pages of description. I was hoping not to run out of ink. And I saw the price tag that would equal roughly a semester of tuition for Weldon. I was bluffing in my question that I knew this is the school he attended.

He didn't blink.

"I make an arrangement to trade out work for tuition," he said, agitated.

I almost jumped out of my seat.

"What is the verification process of his claims?" Bob asked the trustee.

DeMars explained there was no verification process, but he could pursue criminal sanctions if he believed my ex-husband had perjured himself. "He testified under penalty of perjury," DeMars said.

My former husband looked rattled.

"He signed a statement that these documents are true. Child support cannot be discharged," DeMars explained.

It was something I gathered their father did not internalize. And good luck collecting from a man with $300 in reported income from spiritual tourism.

"Be a man, be a father," I told him when he called to wish me a happy Mother's Day the year before. "Words are cheap. The woman at the grocery store wished me a happy Mother's Day, too, and she doesn't even know me. At the very least, be a man and pay the financial support you are required to pay."

"I didn't call to hear this." Then he hung up. He hadn't asked to speak to the boys.

My last round of questions in DeMars's office began when I asked him his name. He sent correspondence now as "Matthew," but he filed for bankruptcy under his legal name. My ex-husband said he changed his name to his middle name.

"You ought to sign your e-mail responses to him with a different name every time," Madeleine suggested. "Barbie," or "Esmeralda," she said. "Whatever you feel like."

His legal name was the same, he explained. But now he preferred to be called Matthew. "Will you call me Matthew?" he asked me.

I shook my head. No, and I won't call you Grumpy or Sneezy or Sleepy either. It's not your name. Your boys' names are still the same.

He asked Bob to call him Matthew.

"Sure, I'll call you whatever you want," Bob answered.

My ex-husband guffawed and whacked Bob a slap on the leg, a little too hard, a little too intense.

"Does Matthew have assets?" I asked. "What is Matthew's income?"

The trustee said questioning was over.

"I am trying to establish that he has an alias," I said. My heart was pounding in my chest.

For goodness sake, he has a new name, doesn't give the right address—isn't that wrong?

The trustee stood up and I shook his hand, thanking him for his help in collecting past child support. He told me it cannot ever be discharged, that he will owe it forever. *And he will likely pay none of it,* I thought.

"Pick a place on the map and we will go there together," he wrote in a card to Colin one year with a picture of a map of the world.

It was all I could do not to circle Illinois and say, here, this is where they live, this is where you can send the check, this was where their lives are, this is where they eat and sleep, study, laugh, and cry. I wanted to add a P.S.: "We don't do much world traveling these days, paying for tuition; food; the mortgage; phone, gas, electric, and medical bills and all. Send the check."

I wanted him to hold up his responsibility because I did not want to spend my money and energy chasing him down. Anyone who has gone through a lengthy divorce and tried to collect on a deadbeat parent knows the physical, financial, and emotional toll such pursuit requires. If he was living in Amsterdam, I could not garnish his wages. If he was without a regular paycheck no matter where he was living, I could not demand a portion of zero. I was out hundreds of thousands of dollars for the boys' future. And he knew it. He could slide away.

It was and it wasn't about the money. It was about being a parent, one who took to heart the ties to his children. I could not excuse the choice to escape. I could not hide from the realization that having a parent deny you would make your heart shatter and the shards would remain.

"Call me on my cell phone," he wrote to Colin. "I pick up messages periodically."

If it wasn't so cruel, I could laugh. What he needed to do was beg for their forgiveness. "I am sorry" is what he needed to write first, not suggest a vacation. "I am sorry I missed it all," was the card he needed to send. "What can I do to make it up to you?" is what he should have written. "I was wrong."

A few weeks later my friend Lillian suggested I write on a piece of paper how much child support he owed the boys, light it on fire, and burn it in the fireplace.

"Let it go," she said. "Give it to the universe."

I felt a little silly, but I did it. In just a few seconds, the yellow piece of paper ignited and transformed into ashes in the living room fireplace. There, I gave it to the universe. Now it was smoke.

What I wanted to say to my former husband was this: Promise to be a father. Let them decide to allow you back in. I could have explained to him that none of the boys wanted to see him right now. That they wanted to be in control of the event if and when they saw him. That they would no longer be passive and let him do what he wanted to them. They would call the shots. I should have told him Weldon's fantasy was to go with me to this hearing this afternoon to beat him up.

"I don't think that's a good idea," I told Weldon.

I could have said Brendan fantasized about how he could pummel him to the ground and make his father cry, that he was big enough now to hurt him, that he was much stronger than his father ever was. I could have said Colin told me he wondered if his dad ever loved him. And that he forgot what he looked like. When I asked him if he wanted to look at old pictures of him, he always said no.

I wanted to tell him that this act of legally disavowing himself from any past, present, or future child support hurt them immensely. It hurt them on a tangible, practical level, and it hurt them emotionally that their father would think this public act to dissolve his responsibility for any of their needs was OK. I wanted to tell him that he could not take back the harm he caused and he could not pretend it didn't happen; it was not OK to assume forgiveness, that everything was excellent, no one was a victim. Forgiveness needed to be earned.

I could have told him that one year when he sent Weldon a birthday card with a photo of himself on it, Weldon tore it into many pieces. I wanted to tell my ex-husband that when he called perhaps once a year and left a message in the middle of the day when obviously no one was going to be home, the boys became infuriated when I suggested someone call him back. And then they turned on me. And that the anger and the fury were palpable in our house for days. It was harder and harder for them to pretend to his family that their father had not abandoned them.

"Stop asking," Brendan said to me. "We don't want to hear about him."

"I am sick of talking about him, never say his name again," Weldon said.

I wanted to tell him they are all good sons. They are smart, loving, and more than any parent could ever dream. I wanted to tell him that Colin is so shaped by his loss that the reason he wants everyone to like him is because his own father does not. I wanted to shout at him that Weldon and Brendan can't trust many people because their own father ran away from them, their needs, and even the sound of their laughter.

I could have tried to say all of it, but I said nothing. It would not have mattered much anyway. There had been too much talk and now too much silence. Nothing was changing. The boys didn't really forget. They harbored the injury; maybe it stayed there forever, maybe they only learned where to compartmentalize it and stop blaming themselves or me for what their father had done.

Bob and I walked to the elevator; my ex-husband was standing inside, the red arrow signaling it was going down. Bob started to get in.

"Bob, you have to be kidding me," I said. Bob stepped back out.

"That's a lot of energy to spend, Michele," my former husband said, holding his wheeled black duffel bag by the long handle.

"Use your energy to write a check for tuition," I said.

The door closed. Bob and I went to lunch at Italian Village just east of the federal building. Upstairs next to our booth was a long center table of eighty Chinese men of middle age—we counted. All were wearing ID tags, all eating the same lunch of spaghetti and meatballs, and later all eating the same naked scoops of vanilla ice cream. I read in the paper the next day that thousands of delegates from Lions Club International were in Chicago for a convention; they must have been Lions.

I had a chicken salad with apples and pine nuts. It tasted like rubberized air. I couldn't smell, I couldn't feel, I couldn't taste. I was numb, but the hearing was over. Hopefully I wouldn't have to go to court for him for another twelve years.

"The poor guy," Bob said over lunch. "He's fifty years old, can't rent an apartment, can't rent a car, can't get a credit card, can't even get a hotel room."

I didn't pity him; his choices had created all of this mess. And his choices hurt the boys. He couldn't hurt me anymore, and I was not scared of him. Maybe I never could protect the boys from his brand of hurt.

Last summer Colin and I were going for a walk after dinner.

"If Dad doesn't call me today, I won't love him anymore," he said. "Maybe he will call tomorrow."

I felt as if the air had left my lungs. Of course he didn't call that day or the next. Or the next. It was another year and a half before Colin would stop waiting for him to call. When I asked Colin if he wanted to see his father after he sent me an e-mail that he was in town, Colin said no. He later told me that with Weldon by his side, he called his dad on his cell phone and left him a message that he never wanted to see him again, that he should leave all of the boys alone.

When he told me the story later that night, I tried not to offer judgment or to say anything bad about his dad. "How did you have his number?" I asked.

"It's the same cell number he always had. It's one of those numbers burned in you that you never forget," Colin said. "His message uses his new name and says he is filled with light or something like that. Do you want to hear it?"

I declined.

"I told him it has nothing to do with you and to stop blaming you. It is him who left us," Colin said.

I spent the rest of the summer writing a book about the trends in storytelling in journalism and getting Weldon ready for his first year of college. Weldon didn't want the blue and white striped washcloths tied with blue ribbon from the back-to-campus section from Target. But I bought them anyway. He said he liked the Buddha plaque I bought on sale for his desk in his room, but he left it in the family room at home when he packed the boxes, and filled the contractor bags with what seemed like everything else he owned. My sister Maureen knitted him an enormous afghan in red and white stripes, University of Wisconsin's colors. He wanted that.

We loaded the white Buick Rendezvous to the roof with a black futon Paul gave him, a side table, desk lamp, suitcases, and the matching plates and cups in red. I moved him—OK, he did the actual moving—into his dorm room in Smith Hall, fifth floor. I filled his refrigerator, neatly arranged his clothes on the shelves in the open closet he shared with his roommate, and made his bed with three comforters, all in matching blues. I bought him a sisal rug with red trim and put the towels on his shelves. He wouldn't let me get more pillows for the futon.

Weldon was a recruited walk-on for the University of Wisconsin–Madison wrestling team and was red shirted, meaning he would practice with the team but not compete. Wrestle-offs for the 149-pound spot were weeks away. Starting immediately he would be going to practice and weight lifting three to five hours a day in the new wrestling room at Crandall Stadium. This was the school he wanted, this was the team he wanted, Big Ten, Division I; he was exactly where he wanted to be.

He had to say no to the private university he would have liked to attend because it was far too expensive per year in tuition and fees. He liked the coach, loved the campus when he had an overnight stay in the spring, but it would be impossible for me to swing it. I thought the head wrestling coach would be the next Powell in his life, and I loved the thought of that. So I felt more than a little guilty about having finances be the main reason he wouldn't go there, but I couldn't incur that much debt for one son for one year of college. I had a conversation with the financial aid office staff, and they demanded to see Weldon's father's tax returns. I tried to explain that was impossible.

"At this university we consider it both parents' responsibility for tuition," the financial aid officer explained.

Weldon's high school dean wrote a letter to the financial aid office saying she had never met the father, he had nothing to do with the boys, he was not involved. My neighbor, who knew the boys well and happened to be a psychiatrist, wrote a letter to the financial aid office and reiterated that I was the only parent involved. Nothing helped.

"Both parents are responsible for tuition," the woman said, when I called to ask if the letters were received. With three sons, I had eleven more tuition years to go. I had to be smart. Weldon was happy with the choice he made. Paul offered to help me with tuition. Working at the university afforded me portable tuition—40 percent—which I desperately needed.

In the summer after seventh grade, Weldon had been to a wrestling camp at University of Wisconsin, stayed in the dorm on the lake, sharing a room with a thick-necked boy who unpacked a case of orange Crush and bags of pork rinds and Cheetos when I dropped Weldon off with his duffel bag.

Just as I did those years before, I knew he would make it; I had faith in him. I could cross him off my daily worry list. He would be fine.

▪ 16 ▪

CLOCK

August–December 2007

The first week of December in 2007 I told my three teenage sons that in three weeks I would be having surgery. I didn't say what for. Not one of them asked any questions. Not one.

The year before was the breast cancer. Here we go again.

I got through that just fine, always wearing my happy, strong face in my sons' presence. "Cured" is what Dr. Dowlat called me, and though I would take medication for at least five more years as instructed, I was going to be fine, 98 percent chance of fine. Which is pretty close to fine. I was not going to die. Not from that anyway.

All the psychology and child development textbooks will confirm this as normal: My three boys were not empathetic or interested when I introduced a new surgery to the calendar. Altruism is not so common in that age range. However, you would have thought they would be just a teensy bit curious. After all, I had been the only parent in the house for twelve years, since Colin was one year old. Their father had been estranged from them for three years at that point.

Weldon was eighteen and a freshman at UW living in a dorm room with a young man who was a musician and who routinely stole his protein bars. The good news was the roommate went home almost every weekend. But during the week, the roommate's friends stayed over in the closet-sized room with the predictable bunk beds; the friends slept on the floor or in chairs. It was not ideal. Save the free bagels in the lobby of the dorm, it would have been miserable.

Brendan was a junior in high school, sixteen, spending his home hours in his man cave in the basement—two TVs, an Xbox, futon, couch, bed with too many mismatched pillows, and a refrigerator around the corner. I moved Colin and Brendan to separate bedrooms when Brendan was ten because I could not survive their shouts and threats to each other—over everything from muddy shoes to push-ups to chicken wings—every night before they fell asleep and every morning when they woke up to fight about toothpaste. It was calmer when each son had his own room.

Colin was thirteen and an eighth grader with Justin Bieber hair he tended to religiously. He rode his bike to school and back—with one friend balancing on the handlebars and another standing on the pegs attached to the back wheels. Of course no one wore a helmet.

How would they know if they didn't ask? It could have been plastic surgery—though I do not believe in it for cosmetic reasons only. I prefer to think I am loved for my mind. I do not lie about my age because I think denying how old you are somehow negates your right to be on the planet. I want to be here and I want each minute I have been here to count, to mean something. Do not erase me, nor the lines on my face or the freckles on my arms.

They didn't ask. I could be having a toe amputated or an organ removed. No one asked.

At dinner more than a week later, Colin did.

"I'm having my ovaries out," I said without emotion or explanation.

Brendan looked mortified. "Gross! You still have those?"

I didn't tell them my doctor thought I had ovarian cancer. I didn't tell them that I was terrified I was going to die. I just kept chewing.

Getting to this point involved a tedious list of unwelcome discoveries—ultrasound to elevated CA-125 test to another elevated CA-125 count on a second test—all leading to the conclusion that I had either benign cysts or ovarian cancer. The nickname for ovarian cancer is the silent killer. As if you would prefer a loud killer.

I am going to die. I didn't die from the breast cancer, but now I am going to die from ovarian cancer. I dodged the first bullet, but not this one; this one is going to get me. This is no cancer lite. It's a death sentence. No one survives. The breast cancer was a dry run. This will do it. This is the real stuff. My children will not have a parent. My children will be orphans. Mothers die.

In my pre-op appointment in her office, Dr. Lauren Streicher said she would go in laproscopically, "disconnect the left ovary"—that was the term she used. I envisioned it as complicated as unplugging the cable to the TV in the basement—remove it, seal it in a plastic baggie, and if it was clearly benign, then the procedure was over.

If the mass was suspicious, a pathologist on call would do a frozen section and Dr. Streicher would have an answer in thirty to forty minutes as to whether or not it was cancer.

Frozen section. Now I am picturing egg rolls, pizza, and spanakopita in the grocery store aisles with the frosted glass doors that open slowly.

If it was cancer.

If it was cancer, she was just going to remove all of it—everything. I pictured my abdomen like an empty shoebox.

"It will take one to one and a half hours tops if there is no cancer. If there is cancer, maybe two hours," Dr. Streicher said, deliberate and poised.

I wrote it down carefully in my notebook.

One hour equals no cancer.

Two hours equals cancer.

I have been to many funerals of mothers—and fathers—and they are always horrific, even the ones where the husband is brave and the bagpipes are playing. Especially those. My two brothers have lost their wives—Madonna had ovarian cancer, Bernadette a brain tumor. My friend Catherine died before her four children were grown, and they each sobbed fitfully at the funeral as her husband nearly collapsed at the podium of the church, thanking everyone for coming, in a robotic voice that sounded like a phone recording at the bank. Sue and I sat together in the neat pews. Cecilia and I drank wine at the lunch. Sometimes I think I see Catherine driving past me on the way to the grocery store in her van. And I think I need to call her. She is dead.

It's no better when the fathers die, but at least with the fathers, there is some kind of hope; that is, if the mother can hold it together. The father dies and no one is thinking the family is completely doomed now, because the mother will hold it together. None of it is good, and the fathers do OK, but it's a peculiar kind of horror when a mother dies; she is often the keeper of the secrets, the soft heart, the timepiece that regulates everyone else. The center of gravity. Everyone loses their footing without her, like quicksand.

Lying on the gurney, before I was wheeled into surgery, my sister Madeleine held one hand, my sister Maureen the other. Mary Pat stood at the end of the gurney.

It was 7:30 in the morning. Of course I had been up all night, the way you are when you are so nervous and when common sense will not land on you. You think if by sleeping you are saying it is normal, this is fine, let's go about our everyday business, shall we? Lying down would be wrong; closing your eyes and surrendering would be unwise. No, you must stay up, stay awake, greet the sunrise, keep vigil soldier sharp over the madness. It is not just another day.

It would be over by 9:30 AM. Either way. I wonder if I should renew my magazine subscriptions. The nurse took my glasses. I couldn't see anything clearly.

Count down from 100.

99, 98, 97, 96.

When I woke up in recovery, I searched for the wall clock, frantically, squinting. There it was, a large white circle with black numerals big as my fist: 9:50 AM. I had been in surgery more than two hours. More than two hours. More than two hours equals cancer.

I was going to die.

Maybe this was how it would be; isn't this how it is for all of us?

I would go along, get on with my life, raise the boys, work, and never really know how it would end up, not at all conscious of the fine-print details on anything. Any degree of certainty was an illusion, self-deception at its worst. There always exists the chance that at any moment any one of us could be pirated by misfortune or someone's capricious change of heart.

Cancer the size of a moth. A decision to walk through a different colored door. A right instead of a left. This flight instead of the next. At any time the cancer could come back. At any time, anything.

I started to cry, a convulsing, sobbing hurricane of tears. I wouldn't see the boys graduate from college. I wouldn't see them get married, have children. And I was so hoping their wives would like me. I wouldn't get to go to Australia, Sweden, Thailand. I wouldn't get to paint more, have a nice kitchen, write more books, love someone so much I could float.

I think as a mother—or father—the second you hold your squirming infant, with tiny hands and soft doll lips, it all stops being about you. You as first anyway. The airline staff need to remind you to put the oxygen mask on yourself first before you affix the mask to your child, because your instincts will not allow you that option.

You pay their tuitions first, you give them the window seat, the benefit of the doubt, the blanket when you are cold, the forgiveness you won't give yourself. Because that is what mothers do. And doing that does not feel sacrificial or martyr-like; it feels normal. To not do that regularly, consistently, and before your first conscious breath of the day feels like a betrayal of who you have become, of who you have been miraculously granted to be.

It is only when you see and understand fully that the door may be closing forever that you wish maybe you had jumped out the window once or twice for a stroll by yourself when the moon was full. It is then that you thrash helplessly in regrets and almosts and never got to's. It is then that you become selfish and demanding and howling angry. It is then that quiet and accepting seems impossibly insane.

Maybe only two or three minutes later, Dr. Streicher, her head covered in a blue surgical cap, walked over to the bed, held my hand and said, "There is no cancer."

I sniffled. "But it has been two hours . . . "

"It all went very well. You have been in recovery for a while."

When I fly—which is about once or twice a month for work—I play this game in my head when the plane is landing; it's kind of morbid, really. The closer we get to the ground in the last few minutes of approach, I think, *if we crashed now, I would not live*. Descending faster, closer to the ground, the stripes on the runway below. *If we crashed now, I could survive*. Wheel touch is imminent. *If we crashed now, I would definitely live*. And then we land. Sometimes the passengers clap.

17

AGAIN

November 2008

I volunteered to make sub sandwiches to sell at the first dual meet of the season. I picked up the ten extralong baguettes from the bakery and went to Costco for the rest of the ingredients. I moved my cart through the cavernous aisles, stopping for sample bites of chimichangas or chocolate truffle pieces offered by smiling hair-netted women with thick ankles. For two youth football seasons I made subs for the Little Huskies home games; all the profit for the team went into helmets and pads for the kids. We always sold out of the subs I packed in coolers marked TURKEY or SALAMI.

The Wednesday before Thanksgiving I worked from home in the morning and then spent about three hours making eighty sub sandwiches—ham, provolone, salami, roast beef, lettuce, and tomato. My hair, my hands, my clothes, everything smelled like a corner deli; the sweet tomato scent mingling with the salty roast beef juice and the spiced aroma from the thin, sweating slices of salami. Caryn came over to help. Two hours into it, I remembered why I never wanted to work in a restaurant as a teenager. From the time I was fifteen,

I worked retail, preferring to sell cheap jeans and trendy T-shirts rather than serve someone food. I stacked the wrapped sandwiches in empty boxes and Weldon helped me get them to the car.

"Leave some for us," Weldon pleaded.

Powell called this first night of the wrestling season the Huskies Alumni/Wrestling Family Reunion, and close to six hundred former coaches and wrestlers, as well as parents, friends, and classmates, cheered from the stands in the field house. Weldon was home for Thanksgiving weekend from school and would be on the sidelines to help coach his brothers through each of his matches. This was Brendan's last season in high school; he was wrestling at 171, moving from junior varsity to varsity at times since the seniors on the team stacked pretty deep at that weight.

The week before Brendan won one wrestle-off match against another 171-pounder for the varsity spot and lost the final wrestle-off for the varsity position. Brendan would be co-captain of JV as a senior, and he was fine with that. Colin was wrestling in his first high school meet at 119 pounds, the same weight Weldon wrestled as a freshman. It was my sixth year in those wrestling stands.

This first night of the season hummed with possibility and anxiety. Tonight, everyone's record was 0–0. As a member of the team, it was exciting to have so many fans, but unnerving; no one wanted to mess up in front of such a big crowd, a crowd easily three times the size of a regular home dual meet.

"It's balls to the walls," Colin said.

The stands began to fill just before 6 PM; parents of former wrestlers waved hello, hugged other parents of wrestlers and alum wrestlers, brothers here for younger brothers. You knew the loss for your son would weigh heavy or the win would make him ebullient. You also knew he would be sore and exhausted and maybe sport a fresh black eye from an errant elbow or a purposeful jab. You would wash the singlet quickly and you would talk late that night with him about the smallest details of the match, second by second it seems, recounting each shot, takedown, crossface, cradle, illegal hold, and referee mistake. And together you would go over not just his match but the match of everyone on the team. And if the team won, you would celebrate.

"Did you see Ellis pin that guy?"

And yes, I did.

Between matches moms chatted about Thanksgiving, who was having what at whose house, making lists of what to buy or bring or cook for the next day.

"I'm not on until Saturday," I reported. That was when my family got together. I was scheduled to pick up a twenty-six–pound fresh turkey the next day. It looked eerily like a sleeping toddler when I unwrapped it and placed it in the enormous roasting pan. I was making sweet potato soufflé for the party at Paul's house.

It was a good thing to have our family Thanksgiving dinner delayed to either Friday or Saturday after the actual Thanksgiving— for years the boys couldn't eat much at all on Thursday; they wrestled on Friday and Saturday and needed to make weight, even with the two-pound allowance for midseason. But it was a tradition started by my mother, decades before there were wrestlers in the family. My mom said she despised the stress of hopping from family to family on holidays with six children in tow, so when Mary Pat married Ken, she declared we would begin a new tradition and have our Thanksgiving on a different night than Thursday.

Both junior varsity teams wrestled first on two mats. Brendan won his match 9–3; Weldon was crouched at the edge of the mat, shouting to him what to do next, cheering him on. Brendan looked strong, dominating all three periods; the only points scored on him were escape points.

"Let's go, B," his teammates shouted.

"Go, Brendan," the parents on our team yelled from the stands.

That is one of the things I loved about wrestling—escape points. You maneuvered out of a hold, you came back from a down position, you got a point. The folkstyle wrestling point system worked the way I wish life did; it was a pragmatic and judicious approach. If your opponent exhibited any of the following sins: unnecessary roughness, unsportsmanlike conduct, stalling, illegal holds, or technical violations, you earned a point. I liked that the competitor's transgressions worked in your favor. In a sense, you were rewarded for not behaving badly, for playing by the rules. And your opponent was punished by you earning points.

You had to keep trying, you had to keep wrestling, no stalling, waiting out the clock or running away from your opponent. That could get you a stalling warning and eventually could earn your opponent a point. If you consistently backed out of a hold or tried to just get the heck out of bounds before you got pinned, you were stalling and your opponent scored. And you must be a good sport. I have watched boys head butt, shove too hard for an escape, head slap, pull on the other wrestler's headgear, or trash talk. They were penalized. If the referee didn't see it, the fans screamed until he did.

It was reassuring to have a traditional, centuries-old sport that regularly monitored civility and proper behavior. Even if it seemed as if the physicality was brutish, there was a higher sensibility and civilized requirement to the sport. The wrestlers shook hands before the match. They shook hands after the match. At the end of the final period, each wrestler went to shake the hand of the opposing coach. Sometimes the wrestlers hugged each other. Colin did this at times; especially if he knew his opponent from youth wrestling.

Nothing personal, sorry I pinned you, it's just wrestling.

The sport accommodated time to bleed; five minutes a match per wrestler.

"You got to love a sport with blood time," said Tom, a father of three wrestlers.

Blood time was the official pause so a trainer could gauze up a wrestler's nosebleed or cut and the staff could wipe down the mats and the other wrestler with antibacterial spray and treated wipes handled with plastic gloves. Up front it was an acknowledgment that you might get hurt and that regulations allowed for some brief medical attention. So you had time to be patched up, the blood wiped from yours or the opponent's arm or leg or face, and you got right back to it.

The referee blew the whistle to stop wrestling for a potentially dangerous hold or a stalemate. Wrestlers couldn't keep hanging on each other in what we sometimes called the heavyweight dance, standing head to head, arms gripping arms, feet slowly moving across the mat. You had to make progress, keep moving. Do something. Stand up. Wrestle. Shoot.

Of course, pinning was the whole point. That was when a wrestler had both shoulders or shoulder blades of his opponent flush to the mat for two seconds. The referee lied flat on the ground, whistle clenched between teeth, inches away from the wrestlers, trying to see if both shoulders were touching the mat, sometimes trying to swipe a hand between shoulder and mat; and if it was not possible—bam—he slapped his hand on the mat and the pin was complete, match over.

You loved to hear that sound if it was your son pinning the opponent or your teammate pinning the other side. It was deafening if the mat pound signaled you were pinned. Your team won the most team points—six—for an individual's pin. So you were not just winning your match, you were propelling your entire team to victory. Pins were good. If you were the pinner, not if you were the pinnee. What I most liked about pinning was that no matter what the score was or had been for the entire match, even if you were losing 14–0, you could pin your opponent and win. A pin trumped the score. There was at every second the possibility of redemption; there was always hope. A pin was also called a fall, and it had a literary Roman gladiator ring to it, like fallen soldiers, fallen heroes, fallen angels. A fall from grace.

You could also get out of a near-pin, maybe not so much a cradle, when your opponent had you chicken-winged and bent, his arms locking you in a hold that had you trapped and immobile. And for that your opponent could earn more points: for a near-fall, three back points earned if he held you there for more than five seconds; two points if he held you for two, three, or four seconds.

"Wouldn't that be awful to be trapped like that?" I said to Caryn at a meet a few weeks later.

We were watching boys other than our sons, and one wrestler had his opponent twisted and bent beneath him in what looked like near suffocation.

"Yes, it would."

But yet no matter the circumstance on the mat, the system was designed to reward effort and enterprise. You could earn two points for gaining control of the match, a reversal; you were down and then you were on top. It was an underdog way of looking at the world. You could win at any moment, no matter the score. There was a limit to a scoring disparity. The wrestling stopped with a fifteen-point lead; a ceiling on the humiliation. You may lose, but you would never be too big a loser. Or too big a winner. It was a system that cushioned for arrogance. There were no ties; a winner must be declared, a decision made, even if it took three overtimes. Someone would win. And someone would lose.

And if it could not be decided in three two-minute periods, there were bonus points—the overtime periods when you could prove yourself again, come back stronger, show what you had. Prove yourself. Change the outcome. Win.

At the end of it all, no matter what the decision, both would leave it on the mat and walk back to the team and take a seat. If you didn't behave properly—say, threw your headgear or stormed off the mat, your team would lose points. And if you did, you would humiliate your coach. It meant your coach did not teach you how to be a good sport. It meant your coach, well, your coach was an ass.

Your coach set the tone of the team. If your coach was a stand-up guy, the entire team was respected. How you behave mattered; it affected everyone else. Powell was respected throughout the country. It seemed every high school wrestling coach around the country knew Powell. A clip of his 1994 high school victory was on the overhead video screens in the arena at state. His interview about what it meant to be a wrestling coach was also on video. When his face came on screen, so many cheered.

When all the JV matches were finished from 103 to 285, the freshman team was seated on the metal team stands dressed in gray-and-blue Huskies sweats. The varsity team burst from the wrestling room above the field house, running down the center stairs to applause and shouts.

"Here they come," parents shouted, standing and applauding.

The orange-shirted wrestlers ran in single file around the blue mat with the orange center circle, each wrestler wearing new orange-and-blue wrestling shoes.

"Go Huskies," we stood and cheered.

It was a corny nod to pageantry, this practice of emerging from the wrestling room like warriors descending from on high to the coliseum. But it was part of what Powell had built, a team of boy-men extraordinarily loyal to their coach, ranked first in the state before the season even began, thirty-first in the country.

Colin was called to the check-in table for his weight class. Colin and the freshman 119-pounder shook hands at the start of the match, both upright. Weldon knelt at the side of his mat, cupping his hands to his face and shouting at Colin what to do. Colin scored two take-downs and back points, winning 7–0 with a pin. The ref hoisted Colin's arm in the air. Five years later, Colin looked so much like Weldon on the mat, wearing the Oak Park blue singlet, the shape of his legs lean and gangly, his strong shoulders, and his tousled blonde hair bursting outside the blue-and-orange headgear. Colin was smaller than Brendan, with his large shoulders and broad back, but they all had the same oval-shaped face, blue eyes, and fair skin. And they all had the same shape legs; and the shape is not the same as mine.

After tonight there would be thirteen more tournaments, invita-tionals, or duals for Colin in the season; fifteen for Brendan. Weldon wrestled when he came to Huskies practices to help Coach Powell. Weldon had quit the Wisconsin team during his first season. The biggest reason was the December of his freshman year he won a prestigious scholarship to study at the University of Oslo and travel throughout Scandinavia for ten weeks—the Viking Scholarship. His wrestling coach advised him not to go; it would interfere with his wrestling, because he needed to practice and wrestle all summer to stay in shape. He needed to wrestle every summer, no study abroad ever.

Weldon called Powell often to discuss it. We went back and forth about it; I would ask questions, Weldon would answer curtly, or he would not answer at all. He quit the wrestling team, the most difficult decision he said he ever made.

"Are you done having your hand raised in the air?" I asked.

"I think so," he said.

I had bought the Badger paraphernalia. Weldon didn't see himself going to the Olympics. As he reminded me, some guys on the team had been four-time high school state champions. He was a high school state qualifier twice, a placer once.

The August after his trip throughout Scandinavia, I was waiting for him at the airport's international terminal. I held high a WELCOME HOME balloon, standing shoulder to shoulder with the dozens of other mothers, fathers, siblings, and lovers of travelers. Moments before Weldon emerged from customs, members of the US Olympic team walked through the crowd, fresh from a flight from Beijing, China. Basketball superstar Kobe Bryant, sporting the Olympic gold medal around his neck, was met by a throng of admirers. Young women in USA warmup suits rushed into the arms of family. We all cheered. Weldon walked into view, and at that moment I loved him so fully I thought I could float. He looked like a man. And he also looked like my little boy.

18

CHAMPION

February 2009

I told Brendan to go to school anyway, in spite of his insistence that he stay home. It was just a sore throat. Second semester senior year was my diagnosis. He had been accepted at four colleges already, and applied for early decision in November because of wrestling season. He had choices; I just wasn't so sure he had an illness.

It was Wednesday so I went to campus for class and Colin and Brendan went to school. When Brendan showed up for practice after his last class period, pale and sluggish, Coach Powell told him to go home and get to a doctor; plenty of kids on the team had strep throat.

"Get the throat swab," Powell told him.

Brendan texted me, "Powell said I should go to the doctor."

"We'll go when I get home from work," I texted back.

Powell was a better mother than me.

We went to the drive-through immediate care site where there was at least a two and a half hour wait. We sat in the stiff chairs against the wall and watched a cooking show on the flat screen at one end of the waiting room as mothers of coughing toddlers and infants looked exasperated and nervous. I smiled at them and they smiled back. I would be back in the same office exactly a week later for Colin, who would have impetigo on his left shoulder from wrestling.

Hours later, the doctor gave Brendan a prescription for antibiotics for what indeed was strep throat and a note that he could not go to school until Friday. Junior varsity conference was Saturday and it would be Brendan's last wrestling event of the season, of his career. I wanted so much for him to have the chance to win there—another set of victories—but I didn't say that because I didn't want him to feel worse. Brendan looked vulnerable and sweet. It was funny how your children turned into cuddly five-year-olds when they were sick; no longer men but melting into softer versions of themselves, the sharp edges gone from their responses, a surrender to their circumstance.

"Will you feel able to wrestle Saturday?" I asked Brendan.

"I'm not sure," he said.

"It's your last time." As if he didn't know.

I let him be, did a load of laundry, put out a can of soup for him on the kitchen butcher block island for the next day, and made sure there were enough leftovers in the refrigerator. There were turkey meatballs and penne. It was enough. He would have all day Thursday and Thursday night to rest. I hoped he would go.

"I'm good, I am definitely wrestling," he said Friday morning as he packed three Clif Bars and two clementines in a paper lunch bag.

He definitely would wrestle the conference on Saturday. Most of his high school years he had Weldon's shadow blocking his view of himself, and I knew he would regret missing the chance to be in first place on his own terms. Colin's freshman conference and Brendan's JV conference were at the same time, miles apart. I would go to Colin's in the morning, and at noon go to Brendan's. I had three more years to watch Colin wrestle, junior varsity and varsity. Besides, scheduling it this way showed Brendan I believed he would win and would be wrestling in the finals up until the end.

Anne picked up Colin before 5 AM to get the bus at the high school; her son Mike was on the freshman team as well. Colin's freshman conference tournament began at 8. He was wrestling at

112 now, the team needed him at the spot, and with the weight and growth allowance at this point in the season he needed to weigh 116. Trimming from 120 to 116 at that age was like picking meat off a boiled chicken. At some point, there was very little left to give up; it was all just bone.

"You taking first today?" I asked Colin as he gathered his backpack and passed me to get to the front door.

"Yes, I'm going to win."

It's one of the many things I loved about Colin. Unapologetic confidence.

"I'm winning, going for first," Brendan texted me after his first match, which he won 2–0.

"How is Colin doing?" Weldon asked when he called my cell. "Do you know how Brendan is doing?"

I updated him and had to strain to hear him over the shouts and buzzer yelps of the gym. Colin won his first 22–10, a major decision. In his next match, I sat on the first row of bleachers just off his mat, apparently the father of the opposing freshman right next to me, his taunts and shouts, "Kill him!" a little more than I cared to hear at such proximity. Paul rushed in during the middle of the match and sat on my other side.

The score was 3–2 in the third period, Colin was up. With only a few seconds remaining, his opponent, who had only scored with two escapes, took Colin down, even though both were clearly off the mat and out of bounds. The referee gave no points at first, and the other coach kept screaming, "Two! Two!" to award his wrestler the two takedown points. The referee then raised his hands for two points for the Lyons wrestler. And the match was over. Colin lost.

Colin was furious; he had expected to win. He walked it off for a while, out of the gym and through the hallways, then retreated to the top row of the stands on the opposite side of the gym with his teammates, away from all the parents, away from me. He wouldn't look in my direction. The father of the boy who beat Colin—an enormous furnace of a man—elbowed me as he gruffly lumbered to his feet from his seat in the stands. I called Weldon to tell him. I left for Brendan's tournament across town.

"I'll talk to him about it," Weldon said.

Colin would later win another match 18–10 and pin another wrestler to take third. Nancy e-mailed me the digital photo of Colin standing on the third-place soapbox, beaming. His final record for his first high school season was 29–10. This was his fourth third place at a tournament. He won the freshman takedown award for the year.

"I could have done better," Colin told me later. "I could have wrestled the whole time, every time."

"You weren't wrestling the whole time?" I asked.

"Mom. No. I mean during a match, sometimes you just stop wrestling. And you can't do that."

You could tell a lot about a person from the way he won—or lost. Some of the young men from dual meets to state tournaments appeared furious only at themselves—like Colin. They shook the hand of the opponent, even embraced him, but were filled with a growling internal dissatisfaction that was almost palpable. Some were enraged at the referee or the opponent or the other coach, and they threw down the headgear or refused to shake the opposing coach's hand at the end of the match. Some swore and were penalized. Some cried. Some pounded the mat with their fists when they bent down to take the Velcro red or green strap from their ankles and placed it on the mat. Some looked despondent and wounded as if this one loss swallowed the entire, unknowable future in one voracious, unforgiving gulp.

"Please get me an energy drink," Brendan texted me.

I stopped at 7-Eleven and bought him two—just in case—on the way to the high school. I missed Brendan's next match when he won by major decision, 16–8. Brendan was on to win first or second. For the championship match, I crouched closer to Brendan near the mat. Brendan looked incredibly strong but tired. Sweat was pouring from him, his skin slick and glistening everywhere; he looked pale but powerful, a gladiator.

What mother sends a son on antibiotics to wrestle all day in a gym? The answer is most wrestling mothers did.

Both wrestlers seemed evenly matched; Brendan had a takedown, plus an escape point. At the start of the third period, Coach Messer started screaming to Brendan, "This is your last two minutes!" The boys on junior varsity all sat cross-legged at the edge of the mat, cheering Brendan on.

"Go, Brendan, go, Brendan!"

"You can do it, you can win!" I screamed.

Both wrestlers scrambling, Brendan landed hard on his left knee; I saw him move sharply and wince mightily. He was injured. It was his knee, something happened to his knee.

It was over. What a bad break, what a shame he got hurt in the last few seconds of his final match of his high school wrestling career. I would talk to him about how great it was that he tried and what a tough break it was that he got hurt. And in my mind I was thinking about what doctors to call and how to fix his knee, and hoping it wouldn't require an operation, maybe just ice for several days and a knee brace. We have knee braces. He can ice here after the tournament; the trainers had ice. I knew about ice. I knew about doctors. Just not from my own experience.

I have never had an athletic injury in my life. I broke my first bones at forty-seven—my left hand and little finger. It was a laundry injury. I was carrying an enormous basket of dirty clothes to the washer in the basement and could not see the ground in front of me. Normally this was not a problem. But one of the boys left the large red toolbox in the middle of the floor a few feet from the washer. I tripped on it, dropped the basket, and braced my fall against the cement wall with my left hand. It hurt so much I sat on the floor in the basement and cried. Went to the emergency room, got an X-ray, they gave me a brace.

I made an appointment with the hand specialist for Monday. The boys offered little sympathy. It wasn't a real injury in their minds; it wasn't like I was wrestling. Weldon prepared a bowl of ice and told me to keep my hand in it for five minutes. Right.

Brendan limped backward and then lunged again, as if he was pushed from some invisible force behind him. He took down the other wrestler and kept him on his back, winning three near-fall back points. The score was 7–5. Seconds were ticking, third period, it was almost the end. And then it was over. Brendan won his final match; sore and still limping, he took his first-place medal standing on the top box, holding the cardboard poster of his bracket and the word *Champion* under his name, a 27–6 record for his senior year, as part of the best high school wrestling team in the state. His was the team that would in a few weeks win the most points at the IHSA individual wrestling finals, with one wrestler each in the first, second, third, and fourth places. And the team that would win first in state a few weeks after that.

When it was all over, I asked Brendan, "Do you want to drive home with me?"

"Nah, thanks, Mom, I want to go with the team."

Powell told Brendan he would be in the varsity lineup for team state a few weeks later in certain matches for the 171 varsity starter.

"I want him to have that feeling," Powell said.

Two weeks later, after giving his knee time to rest and icing it every day, against all his strenuous objections, I got Brendan an appointment with Dr. Peter Tonino, an orthopedic surgeon who specializes in athletic injuries and knees. My friend Sue was a nurse in that practice and helped me get him an appointment, just as she did when I broke my hand and Colin broke his collarbone.

The X-ray showed no bone or ligament damage.

"I need to wrestle in team state Saturday," Brendan told Dr. Tonino in the examining room. It was Tuesday.

"We'll need an MRI to be sure it would be all right," he said. We scheduled that for 10 PM that night. Dr. Tonino would wait until he had the MRI results before he could agree to let Brendan wrestle.

"I know this is important to you now," Dr. Tonino said. "But you have to walk on those knees for sixty more years."

Dr. Tonino's nurse called Wednesday night with the news. "No wrestling Saturday," she said. The MRI showed a meniscus tear and a cartilage break.

An hour later Dr. Tonino called. "He will need surgery in the next few weeks at the latest," he said. "I know you understand he just can't wrestle, he can't risk it." He explained Brendan could go home the same day after surgery, be on crutches for a few days, but would be out of sports for three months.

I called Powell.

"I will talk to him today," Powell said. "He had a great season, wrestled real hard with a lot of heart. I'll make sure he is OK."

"I'm not being a wimpy mom," I told him.

"Oh, yes, ma'am, I know, you've gotten much stronger over the years," Powell said.

That Saturday we all went to team state; Brendan on the bus with the twenty-one–team roster, and me, Colin, Caryn, and Danne, Liam's mom, in my SUV.

A few days before, Caryn ordered a plush Siberian husky online; it arrived the night before we left. It was about two feet tall and three feet long with a curled tail. We called him "Champ." We went to Target to get him a blue T-shirt in the children's section, size 5–6. I sewed the Huskies logo I cut from another T-shirt onto the back. We dressed it with headgear and a blue-and-orange scarf another mom knitted for all the wrestling moms a few years earlier. Caryn bought twenty orange and twenty blue bandanas for the parents to wear or wave in the stands. I bought a custom cake that read CONGRATULATIONS, HUSKIES. I thought inscribing FIRST PLACE would jinx the team. I was prepared to leave the cake in the car if they lost. I bought a tube of blue icing to write FIRST PLACE on it should the team win.

We carried Champ to the stands, after he spent a few miles of the highway with his head sticking out of the sunroof of my car.

"It's a whole new level when the parents start dressing up animals," Powell said with a smirk.

Our team won state. About fifty of us sat in the tidy stadium seats waving our bandanas and holding cardboard signs I made the night before. IN POWELL WE TRUST was one. I screamed and cheered so much I was hoarse. We all were. The boys jumped and hugged each other, passed Champ around, held him high above their heads. I ran to the car with Tom, whose son Charlie was on the team, and retrieved the cake; the security guard let us back in. Coach Giovanetti carefully wrote #1, STATE CHAMPS in blue icing on the top.

Brendan was there on the gym floor with the team. Each member of the team was called to the center of the arena by name and handed a gold medal in the trophy ceremony. Because Brendan did not wrestle, his name was not called. He did not get a medal. I watched him smile, but I knew he was extremely disappointed. He had been injured, he didn't wrestle. I could see why he did not receive one. That was fair.

What I didn't know, and Brendan told me later, is that minutes after the ceremony Powell said to him, "You need this more than I do." He handed Brendan his own team state first-place medal.

"The memories are enough for me," Powell said. Weeks later he had Brendan's name engraved on the team state trophy that stood at least three feet high.

■ 19 ■

STRENGTH

April–May 2009

"Powell is sick." Colin told me when he came home from wrestling practice. "He told all of us after practice he has a bad disease."

I had known for a few days through the wrestling family grapevine that Coach Powell found out after team state in late February, after the wrestling banquet at the end of March, that he was diagnosed with a muscular degenerative disease. He was exhausted, but anybody would be with his schedule. A few parents who knew kept it quiet. We waited for Powell to tell all the wrestlers. I had not told my boys.

"What did he say? How did the boys take it?" I asked.

"Even the kids who say stupid things didn't say anything stupid," Colin said. "No one said anything."

Brendan told me Powell was able to bench press 350 pounds before, and now he could do only half that. He was "gassed," as they called it, not his usual self. Powell's schedule was grueling, but normally Powell never seemed to wear out. He had a biopsy of a section of his shoulder muscles and the results were in. He sent an e-mail to the wrestling family listserv.

I have been diagnosed with polymyositis. Not ALS, not lupus and not muscular dystrophy. Which is wonderful. However polymyositis is no joke. My muscles have and continue to "melt." I have the strength in my major muscles of a small child and I fatigue with very little exertion. I am on severe doses of prednisone and am showing progress. It will be many months before my strength is back. Polymyositis goes into remission for 20 percent of patients and they never suffer symptoms again. The other 80 percent face an ongoing battle. I'm hoping for remission status. Either way, this really sucks. For a guy whose entire, apparently fragile, persona is predicated upon physicality and activity, it is particularly hard to swallow, I should have been an academic.

Obviously my biggest concern is that I will not have the energy to keep the wrestling program going the way we are accustomed. So any and all help is welcome. I am being told not to push myself, which goes against everything I stand for, but I am abiding nonetheless. Thanks for your well wishes. And keep in mind, I'm no punk. My spirit is strong.

In relentless pursuit,
Michael Powell

I talked to Weldon, who had been in touch with a few of the wrestlers from his varsity team. He called Powell immediately.

"Coach Powell looks like a fourteen-year-old boy, Mom," Colin said. "He is so skinny."

The next evening I was driving a few of the wrestlers home after practice. They did not act like they normally did—loud, laughing, kidding each other.

"Coach Powell is real bad," Ellis said.

"What are we going to do?" Jake asked.

At a freestyle/Greco Roman tournament a week later, Powell looked much thinner, his calves the width of broom handles. He walked like an eighty-year-old man—with a cane—and needed a folding stadium chair to sit in as he coached the matches.

"I'm starting to feel better," Powell said. "If all my prayers are answered, this will be OK."

I asked him if the parents could pitch in and get him a dog walker. He said no. I asked him if we could get his meals delivered. He said no. I asked him if he and Elizabeth needed a housekeeper, and he said he had one. I asked him if we could go grocery shopping for him.

"No, I want to do as much for myself as I can," he said. "But thanks."

"For goodness sake, you have held us all together and helped us raise our kids," I wrote him later in an e-mail. We all wanted to do something. But what we had to do was wait.

"It has and always will be my honor to have coached Weldon and Brendan (and now Colin)," Powell responded in an e-mail to my own message of thanks.

Powell went to Akron, Ohio, with the off-season team for a regional wrestling championship. He went downstate with the team for a freestyle/Greco Roman state tournament, where Colin competed. Powell continued to plan for the off-season; he was the soul of the team. The weekend before Mother's Day, Powell sent an e-mail to everyone on the wrestling families listserv. It read:

As many of you know, I am sick. My immune system is attacking my muscles and destroying them at an astonishing rate. I've lost thirty pounds of muscle. My energy level is probably 15 percent of a healthy person. Current strength is less than my five-year-old neighbor, who carried my groceries in for me the other day. Mine is a particularly aggressive case (Huskie style).

It's been an interesting couple of months. The week after we won the state championship, I declared my life to be the greatest in the world, as I could not imagine feeling better about things. Unknown to me, the extreme fatigue I was experiencing was not due to exhaustion from the long season. Instead, it was at this time that my symptoms began to surface. Weeks later, unable to bench press the weight I did in eighth grade, I dragged myself into the doctor's office.

There was plenty of inner debate about whether or not to make this public. Certainly, I am not one for drama and pity parties. Nor do I wish to have people bringing pot roast over, as I am fiercely independent and have an overdeveloped sense of pride. . . . It is important that the wrestlers see that courage in the face of adversity is not just something the coaches preach, but live. It is important that the wrestlers see me beat it. It is important that they realize the discipline and spirit that it will take to beat it was learned from our great sport. . . .

I often give the same talk to a wrestler who comes off the mat, win or lose, and has not given everything he had: There are only a few things in this world that you truly have control over. Integrity, courage, and pride are things that we, the Huskie wrestlers, hold dear. Win or lose, regardless of circumstances (bad calls, opponent's strengths, injury, pressure from a big match), you always should expect the highest levels in regard to yourself. You're not going to win every match, or every battle in life. But you can bring integrity, courage and pride, and that is something that can never be taken from you.

Of course my sons' lives have included so much more than wrestling. But there was no single endeavor that meant more to them as boys and as young men. And I was down on my knees grateful that they found this to fill them up; believe me, I knew the possible alternatives. The sport itself taught them rules, discipline, and humility. It taught them to know that most encounters produced a winner and loser, and that there was logic to the equation of action and consequence. And that the start of every match produced new possibilities. Effort led to desired results. Lift weights and you would be stronger. Eat well and you would be leaner. Pay attention to your coach and you would wrestle smarter. Go to the wrestling room every day and you would have a battalion of friends who relied on you and respected you, and you would have coaches to respect and emulate. Work your hardest evenly throughout the match and if you get bonus time, pull out all the stops.

The boys also learned about uncontrollable factors—injuries, bad referee calls, rotten timing, illness—all converging into the mercurial serendipity that produced the end game. It was Powell who taught them to internalize all of it. He was the most important man in their lives, and he was a good man. He was teaching them lessons of true strength.

And for my sons, Powell was a good man in their lives every day. Their own father had disappeared, and this unlikely hero took up residence in their lives and in their hearts. I was not enough for them, I would never be enough. I was not who they wanted to emulate.

For all of the young men on the team for the last several years, they wrestled because of Powell, for Powell. It was the family that he built who needed to return the favor.

Part Four

OVERTIME

■ 20 ■

VISIT

February–March 2010

I was back at my desk following an hour lecture to a group of about sixty university freshmen, at least a dozen of them not paying attention. The first week of any quarter you could spot the students who didn't care so much about the class; they didn't take notes, they didn't ask questions, sometimes they ate lunch during lecture and chatted with each other, like they were sitting at the movies or something. Some passed notes back and forth. One young woman always played with her hair.

No matter what quarter it was or what course I taught, I always felt sorry for the parents of some students. They took out loans, mortgaged the house, did everything they could to pay tuition, to make sure this child had everything needed to succeed, from mini-refrigerator to laptop to tins of homemade cookies. I could picture the tear-filled drop-off at the dorm or overpriced apartment with the new sheets and towels, the plastic Target dishes in the school colors, the suitcases filled with outfits earnestly bought that the kids would never wear. And the parents dragging bags and bins and boxes onto elevators or up narrow stairs, wearing the school T-shirts, the students anxious for them to go home. I could almost hear the parents arguing at the dinner table about what would get postponed because tuition was due. And here were some students doodling in class, or arms folded across their chests, or asleep—impenetrable. And their parents would never know.

My office phone rang. "How fast can you get here? Colin needs to get to the hospital right away," the high school's athletic trainer said after introducing himself.

"What's wrong?" In the seconds before he responded I pictured the worst possible outcome—Colin's neck broken, an arm hanging awkwardly, him lying on the floor motionless; can't help it, it's what I do.

"He has an infection on his leg, and it's warm to the touch. I drew a circle around it, but you need to get him to the hospital."

The red mass was spreading past the indelible black marker circumference drawn on Colin's right leg along with the time: 3:00. It was probably MRSA, the acronym for methicillin-resistant Staphylococcus aureus. And if it accelerates, it is dangerous, really dangerous. Because MRSA does not respond to most antibiotics, unchecked an infection of this type can rage out of control quickly, become systemic, spread to your organs. Kill you. There's a reason people start to freak out at the mention of MRSA.

The wrestlers get it from the mat, each other, or close contact with both. Weldon had it at least three or four times, on his leg, his back, his arm. Brendan once. It starts small, a bright red spot the size of a dime, which looks different from ringworm or impetigo. The wrestlers get that too. But with antifungal cream, ringworm and impetigo go away quickly, in a few days.

MRSA requires an immediate trip to the dermatologist. You have to go after it right away, can't wait, can't let it get better. Because it never does without swift intervention.

With MRSA, patients are prescribed the right kind of antibiotics— Bactrim works—advised not to share towels at home, and told to cover the site. The dermatologist we go to on North Avenue always sees the boys quickly after I call; sometimes he fits one of them in between other booked appointments. He's a much older gentleman—his certificate on the wall from medical school is from the 1930s—and he wears a snug knit cap in the winter and thick goggle-like lenses in all seasons. He usually flirts with me and always jokes with the boys that they should take up chess. Wrestling is bad for the skin.

You can't wrestle with MRSA; you can't pass the skin inspection before the tournament or dual meet. Weldon's infections were never more than the size of a quarter and never interfered with his competing; they cleared up before the matches. But they worsened quickly. In a day an infection could grow deep and look like a red, blue, and black plastic relief map. In the nursing home, my mother contracted MRSA at the wound site on her leg where the doctors extracted veins for her bypass surgery. It wasn't the cause of her death, but it didn't make her any better. In small amounts, MRSA is manageable. It's in your nostrils in microscopically small amounts, it's on all the wrestling mats. Every sport battles with the contamination. Some sports more than others.

I knew exactly what the trainer was talking about, and now I was really mad at myself. The boys are always accusing me of mother hysteria, always telling me to chill, always saying it will be fine with some ice or some heat or some something. They say they are not wimps. But my instincts usually are spot-on. So I was furious that I allowed Colin to do his man-up routine and tell me it was a bump, and I didn't know about athletics and injuries, and I am not a wrestler. And now because I listened to him and not myself, he could really be in trouble.

The week before, Colin had placed first in regionals, wrestling varsity as a sophomore at 119 pounds, winning all his matches. That Saturday I had a 5 PM flight for a business trip to San Francisco, so I could watch him wrestle until 2 PM before leaving for the airport. I was co-leading a convening of The OpEd Project at Stanford University. I had started giving seminars, conducting workshops, and leading fellowships in thought leadership that year. It was remarkably rewarding work, and I could do it in addition to my university teaching load. I *needed* to do it in addition to my teaching load; I was paying for college for the next seven years, many of them double-tuition years for the boys.

I had watched Colin win his first two matches, but I had to leave before the match for first place. But he won it, and Caryn texted me the photo of him beaming on the winner's stand.

The following Saturday was sectionals. Colin was not doing well and did not place in the top three. He placed fifth, so he did not make it to state. Since sectionals, Colin's calf had a red mark that looked as if it was left over from a slap or a slam on the mat. The boys were usually pretty banged up after tournaments, like prizefighters, sometimes with split lips or scratches, or black eyes from an errant elbow. Colin and Coach Powell both thought it was a shin bruise; I urged Colin to ice it. By Sunday it was a bump the size of a golf ball and wasn't receding. It didn't start as Weldon's MRSA encounters did, not with the small red mark. Still, I knew it was odd.

"Let's get it checked out at the drive-through doc," I said Sunday afternoon. That's what we called the immediate care center a few blocks away.

Colin didn't want to go. Coach Powell said it would be fine. The trainer looked at it Friday. I didn't see it on Monday; he was icing it and said it was getting better when I asked. It wasn't.

Now it was Tuesday and the size of an eggplant—dark, purple, and otherworldly looking, like he had swallowed a mango and it showed up whole on his leg. That's what can happen with MRSA; the site fills with the infection because the contents are so toxic and aggressive. This is one of the reasons that hand sanitizers are available throughout hospitals now. There are no hand sanitizers in wrestling rooms.

"I'm an hour away," I told the trainer. "I'll get there as fast as I can." It was a little after 3 PM.

I rushed down the hall to one of the lab classrooms where Caryn was teaching a section of the Multimedia Storytelling class, the lab for the lecture I just finished. We carpooled and I was hoping she could leave with me right away. Her students were working on an assignment, and she could keep in touch with them by cell phone and e-mail. Class would be over in another fifty minutes.

I walked into her class, apologized to the students, and asked if she could be ready to go.

"Colin has to get to the hospital," I whispered to her.

She was in my office in less than four minutes. Traffic wasn't as congested as it usually is; sometimes the trip takes close to two hours door to door. I dropped off Caryn at the high school where her two sons, Ben and Sam, were waiting. Caryn and I laughed at how long it takes just to get home.

"We could be in Michigan by now. On the beach," I said.

Colin got in the car. He looked worried, which was rare. We got to the emergency room at Loyola University Medical Center in another twenty minutes. The entire ride I kept telling him it would be OK, and yes, that next time he should listen to me when I say we need to go to the doctor.

When I said "MRSA" to the triage nurse, everything moved pretty quickly compared to our other ER visits for Colin—the broken collarbone, the chipped elbow, the time Brendan dared Colin to swallow a nickel and he did. Still, we sat in the waiting room for a half hour or so. I texted my friend, Sue, an orthopedic nurse at this hospital; she was still at work at another end of the building. I texted Paul.

A dozen or more patients were sitting in the green plastic and metal chairs in the ER waiting room, including an eight-year-old girl encouraged by her mother to practice her recorder. Everyone with a child in elementary school has had to listen to the scales crucified on that cheap plastic flute. But this would not be a good time to practice. Every sick and anxious person cringed—the older Asian couple, the young Hispanic woman with the two-year-old child in her arms, the woman with the piercing in her nose. No one had the nerve to be direct, though we all gave each other eye-rolling smirks.

Colin politely asked the mother to have her child stop.

"No one wants to hear that right now," he said.

She balked.

"Don't you think my daughter plays beautifully?"

"It's beautiful, but everyone in here is sick."

The mother gave Colin a dirty look. The little girl remained quiet and a few others thanked Colin and smiled at him.

Colin and I were ushered back into a curtained "room," and soon after the doctor saw Colin, he admitted him for overnight intravenous antibiotics and observation. It was very serious.

"What do you need me to do?" Paul texted.

I walked alongside the bed as an attendant rolled Colin to the pediatric floor, all five feet ten inches of him. When the doors opened, a plastic statue of Ronald McDonald greeted us. The halls were brightly colored, with large alphabet block letters on the floor. There was a central nurses' station, and a family kitchen area to one side. It was very quiet, just after 6 PM. Once Colin was in a room, the nurse started the drip for intravenous antibiotics. Colin asked for a sandwich; the staff obliged. Then he asked for two more. He wouldn't need to make weight and he was starving.

The doctors later lanced the wound, which was extremely painful for Colin in spite of the morphine and the local anesthetic shots he received. From the abscess site, the doctors extracted about ten cubic centimeters (cc)—equal to about a cup—of pus and blood. Colin took a video of the process on his phone. I told him not to put it on YouTube.

"You think I want this to be associated with me the rest of my life? I'd be the MRSA guy."

I walked down the hall to the family galley to get a glass of water or tea. A young woman about thirty was also in there, pouring herself a glass of juice. We smiled at each other and exchanged kindnesses, the way you do when your heart is softened by circumstance.

She told me her son had been there a week. I didn't ask her why. She said the hard part was that she had younger children at home and she had to keep shuttling them to relatives, worrying about where they were each day. She looked tired.

I felt lucky.

Weldon began his life in pediatric intensive care. He was premature, born at thirty-seven weeks from induced labor, and his lungs were not fully developed. He was released in a week, but anyone who has had a child in a similar situation knows that while you are there, watching, waiting, your world shrink-wraps around your child, that hospital, those doctors, those nurses. There is nothing more important than what happens moment to moment in that universe. Your concentration is adrenaline-charged, and all you can think about is how fast you can get your child out of there, how soon it will be over and just be a story you tell to friends.

You feel selfish when you watch the parents who cry in the hallways or push children past in wheelchairs; or when you peek in open doorways, adults huddled around a small figure in a bed, tubes and machines accessorizing the scene, balloons with teddy bears and smiley faces bouncing in the artificial wind from the vents. You want them all to get better. You want them all to go home and be fine. But you know they all won't, they can't, and then you pray that your child does get better quickly, that your child doesn't stay, that if there must be a choice, let it be your child who leaves fine—gosh, did you say that? This makes you feel small. And no matter how kind the nurses are—and they always are—and how many times they smile and reassure you, you never want to see them again, ever. You never want to come back. And it makes you feel reckless to feel this way; it makes you feel shallow. It makes you question what gives you the right to expect it all to go well all the time. It makes you question why it never goes well for some—not just for children in other parts of the world dealing with violence, war, hunger, poverty, and disease. Because you know children die in your suburb. They get sick, have tumors, have cancer, get in car accidents, overdose on drugs. You know you are lucky. Some children die. And that's just one reason you cry when you walk back into the room.

The hospital halls were empty this night. The pediatric floor was on lockdown, the nurse explained. Only parents can visit after visiting hours, a brief window that had already passed.

Coach Powell called my cell phone. He wanted to visit Colin and said he would be there later in the evening. When I told Colin Coach Powell was coming, he was elated.

"Really? He's coming to see me?"

"You'll have to say you are his father; only parents can visit," I told Coach Powell on the phone. I explained what door to use to enter after-hours and what room we were in.

At about 9 PM, after practice, Coach Powell walked in the room; the doctor was checking in on Colin again. They chatted about Colin's leg and about wrestling.

"We'll take good care of your son," the doctor said to Coach Powell.

None of us corrected him.

I slept on what the nurses called a bed; it was a windowsill, really, with a one-inch foam mattress in a vinyl covering, the width of my laptop and only about six feet long. I wondered how taller or larger parents could fit. But it was the first time I could be there for Colin without worrying about the other boys or having to call someone to pick up another son, stay at the house, or make sure it was all fine while I was here. Weldon was in Madrid; Brendan was away at school. Colin made jokes; even in the hospital on IV antibiotics, his leg throbbing and sore, he made jokes. We watched a movie, *Back to the Future*.

Colin didn't get better quickly. After that overnight stay, we went back to the hospital to have the wound checked, and it was relanced the day after he was released. It seems the doctors didn't get all the infection out. They didn't give us the right antibiotics, so we needed to switch, and it took another week for the wound to start healing properly and for Colin to start to feel healthy again. MRSA invades your system so you feel tired, rundown, and out of sorts. The doctor told him to eat lots of protein. And rest.

Because he didn't qualify for individual state, Colin did not get to go with the team to Champaign, Illinois, where his teammates, Chris and Nick Dardanes and Sammy Brooks, each won first-place medals. Benny Brooks took third. Charlie Johnson and LaQuan Hightower were contenders. Colin had to keep his leg elevated with warm compresses. Sitting in the cramped stands for two days would make him even sicker.

Caryn texted me all the updates on our team's wrestlers. Colin was on the phone with his teammates.

Colin missed wrestling in team sectionals the next Tuesday, where Oak Park prevailed. He was hoping he could be well enough to wrestle at team state in Bloomington the following Saturday. That was his goal. But he wasn't; he never could have passed a skin test. The scar was still puffy and paler purple, but odd. By the time team state rolled around, the scar was scaling and still red. Coach Powell told him not to rush it; he had two more years to wrestle. Two more years for individual state and team state.

Colin wrapped the wound—now scaly and discolored, though flattened—and went to team state on the bus with the team. We lost to the team from Minooka, Illinois. Coach Powell talked to the boys, many of whom were extremely distraught. And like he always does, Coach Powell gave them perspective.

I drove home with Brendan, who was home from school, and Liam's mom, Danne. Brendan was on the phone with one of his teammates from the 2009 team.

"What did Coach Powell say to the team?"

"I didn't get to hear it," Brendan said. "But I bet it was really great."

It was a good season. Colin had won first in regionals. I was proud of him. I brought a sheet cake with me to Bloomington for the team to share if we had won first place, as we did the year before. Last year we ate the cake as champions. This year I was careful with the wording on the cake, not wanting to be arrogant or presumptive. I kept the cake in the car.

CONGRATULATIONS FOR A HUSKIES STYLE YEAR, I had the woman at the bakery write on the cake in orange and blue.

After we got home from Bloomington, I put the cake in the freezer. We would use it at the wrestling banquet; it wouldn't go to waste.

◼ 21 ◼

BACK

September–October 2010

On this Thursday September morning, Colin chose the gray suit with the thin blue stripes that he wore to his homecoming dance in his sophomore year. That was last year, and standing on the square platform while the chatty tailor chalked the legs and coat, Colin looked tall and thin, still with a little boy's face on a man's body. The tailor on Oak Park Avenue with the thick Greek accent called me "Mrs. Weldon" or "dear," depending on whether or not he was looking at the receipt.

We sat in traffic court waiting for the judge to arrive, a few minutes before 10:30 in the morning. Colin was summoned here for a speeding ticket he had gotten a month earlier for driving ten miles over the limit in a school zone on our street a block from our house. We sat stiffly purposeful and apologetic in the first wooden pew; each row was crowded with teenage boys, mothers, a few fathers, and some nervous young women dressed in clothes too tight, colorful, and revealing for the sobriety befitting a courtroom.

A neighbor of my sister Maureen slid beside me. She was here for her own son's traffic ticket. "Your ex-husband moved back to

189

Chicago, did you know?" she said crisply. "He called the house, it was odd. He's working in the city as an attorney. Been here a while."

I couldn't answer right away; I felt as if the wind was pushed out of me.

Colin overheard and immediately tensed, began tapping his foot. I didn't react to her, though I wanted to shout. I asked a few questions about where he was working and living, thinking, *OK, maybe now I can get some of the tens of thousands of dollars he owes in child support, now that he is in this country. Support plus five years of college tuition and expenses. Half of all food, clothing, and hospitalizations; his part. The father part. The part he completely forgot.*

If the revelation at this moment had not been so bizarre, I would have chuckled at how random it was to learn he was back in the same city—our city. I would not have known. My former in-laws had stopped inviting us to any family events about a year earlier; a round of graduation parties had passed and nothing since Christmas 2009 came our way. Some of my former in-laws sent Christmas cards, but nothing personalized or signed; I gather we were just on some computer-generated list.

Even though the boys' aunt lived a few blocks away, there was no communication from that side of the family. Their only grandparent, their father's mother, had not called the boys in close to a year. She sent us Christmas cards. I thought about my own mother, who even in the months of hospital stays, always asked me to bring the boys with me, had snapshots of them in her wallet, and would bring out photos of her twenty-one grandchildren for anyone who cared to see. Perhaps the freeze from the in-law side was in preparation for their father's return. Who knows. I stopped being polite and accommodating, stopped forcing the boys to attend events on that side of the family. More than six years had passed since their father left, and so much had happened since he dropped off all his belongings in the front hall for the boys to save for his return. The boys had grown to men since Weldon had thrown away everything that was his.

I was tired of being polite.

I could see in Colin's face the hurt; he was blanched. He was a wonderful young man, always tried, was accommodating and pleasant, and everyone who met him liked him. And his own father did not know.

"I am a good son," Colin said.

And my heart almost shattered.

A few minutes later I recognized a friend's husband—an attorney—as he walked to the desk to the left of the judge's bench. I waved nervously.

He walked over to us.

"What's your plan for the ticket?" he asked, leaning toward me.

"Pay the fine?" I answered. It had been more than fifteen years since I had gotten a speeding ticket and was totally out of practice.

"Give it to me."

He took the manila folder that I had neatly marked COLIN'S TICKET with the letter concerning the court appearance information inside. He sat at the desk, filled out a form, spoke to the prosecutor, and in a few minutes we were standing before the judge with the order that the speeding ticket be dismissed if Colin completed ten hours of community service within thirty days.

I thanked my friend's husband.

"No problem. I was here for another kid."

When I got to work later that day, I e-mailed Coach Powell about the sudden reappearance of the boys' father and warned him that Colin was extremely upset.

"Thanks, I will talk to him today," Powell wrote back immediately.

I called Paul. I called Weldon. I called Brendan. I called Madeleine. I worried.

"I'll call Colin," Weldon said.

"It doesn't bother me as much," Brendan said. "He was never all that nice to me." And then Brendan chatted about his new roommates and the four-page paper he had due in a few weeks.

I know, as clearly as I know that hydrogen and oxygen make water, that their father's decision to completely opt out of their lives has changed them. It is as startling a contrast as one between a *before* picture and an *after* picture, the effects of their father's choice altering them as distinctly as radiation, silently changing who they are. And his absence changed me. When you witness a car wreck by the side of the highway, with the ambulance sirens screaming, for damn sure you drive more carefully on the way home. You take no risks, you thank God you are here at all, and you do what you must to keep everyone safe.

I am not a perfect parent, and I am not a martyr. I did what I had to do. And I would never leave my boys.

A few weeks later, on Halloween weekend, Coach Powell, Caryn, and I drove eight of the team's wrestlers to Preseason Nationals at the University of Northern Iowa in Cedar Falls. Powell drove four boys in his black SUV with the license plate, OP WRSTLR. Caryn and I followed behind Powell in her blue Chevy Suburban, roughly the size of my first studio apartment. Two other wrestlers plus Colin and Caryn's youngest son, Sam, were with us. We packed turkey sandwiches, apples, oranges, and Gatorade.

The boys were irritable, passing packets of gum back and forth on the five-hour-plus sun-filled ride, mostly because they all needed to make weight at 6 PM. Colin was down to 135 pounds and couldn't afford to gain an ounce. Sam was hovering at 171, where he needed to be.

After weigh-ins about 8 PM that night, we went to A.J.'s, a local restaurant near the motel with a fish fry and deep-fried everything, a bar with high stools, and waitresses who were confused by how to accommodate a party of eleven, eight of them famished young men.

Powell talked about his health and his fatigue, and said that the next year would likely be his last season coaching. He seemed to be doing better. At least he wasn't sliding any further downhill.

"I can't keep doing this, but I'll stay for Colin and Sammy," he said to Caryn and me.

Powell was still down about forty pounds since his diagnosis, not the robust young man I first met in 2004. Still, he looked healthy;

thin but with good color. He had been strict with his diet and chemotherapy regimen, trying to get enough rest so he could coach. He was trying to push his body into remission. Powell said he and his wife wanted to start a family and because of his heavy doses of medications and the genetic nature of his autoimmune disease, they were looking into adoption.

"I really want to be a father," he said.

For my sons, he had been.

The next day Caryn and I sat in the purple-and-yellow stands of the Unidome for more than fourteen hours. There were twenty-five mats with simultaneous wrestling of fifteen hundred youth and high school wrestlers from several states and more than sixteen hundred matches in all. Colin won two matches and lost two, so he was eliminated and did not place. Sam won the national championship at 171 pounds, five wins, the last over a wrestler from Minnesota he had lost to in earlier national tournaments. We screamed and cheered and took pictures, so heart-bursting proud of our own winner.

That night we drove to IHOP to celebrate, the boys ordering pancakes, chicken sandwiches, milkshakes, and cheeseburgers. When the bill came, Coach Powell passed it to the boys, eight of them sitting at two tables next to ours.

"Look at what you ordered and add 15 percent to it, then give me that money," he said calmly. Then he explained how you arrived at 15 percent. "Tell me how you do that, Chris," Powell said.

The boys looked confused. They passed the bill one to the next, pulling single dollar bills from their pockets, loose change clanging onto the table. This took about fifteen minutes.

"They don't have enough," I said to Powell.

"Oh, they never do," he said. "They are always at least thirty dollars short. But it's good practice."

Powell collected what the boys handed him, then pulled money from his own wallet and paid the bill, leaving a large tip.

It's what we professors call teachable moments.

"No worries," I tell students who e-mail or visit my office with questions about a quiz, deadline, or grade. "You're upset by the small things. Stop focusing on the lint on the car seat. We are on a cross-country road trip so look out the window. Enjoy the view."

Caryn and I met Powell and the boys for the free breakfast in the lobby of the Fairfield Inn the next morning. It was a bright blue October Sunday, and we loaded the trucks with the overnight bags and wrestling gear. Four boys slept in the middle and third seats behind Caryn and me, their mouths open, hooded sweatshirts pulled over their heads. We drove behind Coach Powell on a two-lane stretch through Iowa, past Masonville and Lamont, Backbone State Park, and into the rolling postcard-perfect hills of Galena, Illinois, just over the glistening Mississippi River, headed straight toward home.

22

BLEACH

January 2011

took off my coat and placed it next to my gray purse on the conveyor belt at the security entrance. I hate this government building, the Daley Center, more than any other place in the world, more than the dentist's office with the chatty hygienist who asks me questions while cleaning my teeth, more than the air safety vehicle emissions testing place you only have to visit every few years, more than a dirty ladies' room off the tollway that smells of retching and beer.

I hate that I am headed to the eighth floor; divorce court is there. I am sixteen years past my divorce and the pleadings and filings and appearances and objections and horror that devoured so many days and so many months and so much of me, that it has taken all my strength to move forward and away from the memory. All that work to make the details and specifics stay in the background, grow so small, so distant, and so unimportant to who I am now and what I do and what I believe and how I feel that they disappear, vanish.

The woman in front of me is short and wide, and her cotton-candy, orange-yellow hair lies in thick, bedraggled clumps down the middle of her back. Her eyes are heavily drawn with dark blue shadow—midnight blue would be the Maybelline name—and her cheeks are colored with clownish circles of rouge. She scowls as she places her hooded sweatshirt coat on the metal lane to pass through security. Another woman behind me is talking on her cell phone loudly, and the uniformed officer tells her to put her phone in the smudged plastic container *now*. Cell Phone Woman with the ratted hair—hers in a brunette updo—ignores the security guard and keeps talking. I am afraid there will be a fight or an arrest or a scene. That would be just perfect.

I am headed to the Chancery and Domestic Relations Clerk's office in Room 802. I retrieve my coat and purse from the conveyor belt and dash to the elevator; it is crowded with lawyers in ill-fitting suits, carting beaten cases bulging with files, and men and women staring ahead. No one smiles.

I am here because I am going to finally do what I should have done years ago. Now that my boys' father is back in Chicago and working—I have confirmed—I am going to attempt to retrieve years of child support. Hundreds of thousands of dollars. My stomach feels now as if it is somewhere above my rib cage, and I try to act like I am not drowning in all the unhappiness, all the sordid details of who did what to whom, all the shame and the fault and the pain, the long-ago hurts.

Domestic Relations File Request, that's where I need to go, to read through the files I requested from storage. My copies of the divorce files were destroyed in the basement flood at my house last summer, soaked through. I had to throw them away. I took that as a good sign—finally getting rid of the weight of those years, that divorce that was so much time and money and hurt. Dirty, ruined, gone.

Because my former husband was in Amsterdam for all those years, I could not pursue what he owed. He tried to make the debts all go away with his bankruptcy filing, but even the mediator reminded him he could not. But he was back in the States, in our town, and it was time for me to act. His LinkedIn profile stated he was working as an attorney and offered consulting in life balance. It was surreal what he claimed, but I needed to do my part now, not let him slither away forever. I needed to stand up to him and what he did.

I learned I needed the files before anything could happen. I needed to know the dates, I needed copies of the documents, his filing for abatement of all child support. And I found it all, the motion to stop paying for the boys when Colin was eleven, Brendan fourteen, and Weldon sixteen. I needed to see the exact dates of his requests for extensions and new dates for a pretrial—ten to be exact—and I needed to see the date in 2006 when I stopped my pursuit, stopped paying for an attorney to pursue him and stopped pretending it was worth my time or my energy to fight him anymore.

The woman at the counter for Domestic Relations File Request is kind, and I am trying to act nonchalant and congenial, like I am at Nordstrom Rack asking for the matching single to a shoe in pink imitation snakeskin. I tell her the file number, she asks my name, and I say, "Weldon"—and then I tell her again that my name and the name on the file are different. She does not seem bothered or confused. The file has my former husband's name and she nods because I am sure she hears this all the time. Women know to lose the former husband's name as soon as they can, that is, if they ever took his name to begin with. She just smiles and asks for my driver's license, and I decide I am going to tell her I am dying inside. I have to tell someone right now because I feel like I am going to implode.

"I cannot believe I am back. I never want to look at these papers again."

"Honey, no one wants to be here." She hands the bulky file to me and I almost wink back because I feel soul-deep relieved that I managed for the fifteen seconds of our pleasant exchange not to want to cry.

I take the cardboard accordion file from 1995 that is six or seven inches deep and head to one of two long, old wooden tables where a half dozen people—mostly lawyers, I gather, because no one looks personally involved and no one looks like he or she is about to cry— and I start to handle each paper. Looking for what I need to copy.

Reading through it all. It strikes me that even the pages have an energy, and I don't want to hold them in my hands because it all comes raging back—the deposition transcripts and the motions and the orders and the different versions of agreed orders—and it is all I can do to take out what I need and get to the copy machine. I have about one hundred pages in all. I have about forty dollars in singles; my attorney warned me the copy machines takes quarters and singles. *I am going to go to the copy machine and copy all these papers and get out of here and never come back. I can do this. I can do this. I never will come back here again.*

I am at the copy machine for so long—maybe an hour and a half or more—that there is a line of people behind me waiting to make their copies. I try to make small talk with a woman in a sweat suit and a baseball cap who is waiting for me to finish.

"I am sorry, I will be done shortly. And I hope never to be in this place again," I say to her. I smile. I want to smile.

I don't think she hears me, but it is too pathetic to say again. I am desperate to be liked, I am desperate to transcend, I am desperate not to feel this gnawing, eviscerating mixture of pathos and anger. I want to cry so badly with every single dollar bill or coin I put in the ancient Xerox machine at twenty-five cents a copy. And I keep pressing copy, copy, copy, copy over and over again as I lift the pages I have separated from the file and put them on the smudged and grayed glass screen, place the cover down, and start again. The copier moves slowly, slowly, slowly with a buzzing, monotonous assertion, like an old man smacking his lips next to you on the bus.

You're back again. You're back again. You're back again.

Everything I touch has a film of dirt and grease, and so many people are walking in and out as if this is just a Dunkin' Donuts or an Arby's. There must be seventy-five people in this area, going through documents, asking for documents, looking for proof, looking for answers, proving what they should already know to be true.

I see my friend, Joni, a lawyer who worked with me on a board of a nonprofit. She looks confused.

"What are you doing here?" she asks. "Did you get married again?"

And then I tell her.

I put back the file, but not before I think really hard about taking the documents and burning them or shredding them to pieces, so maybe that will mean none of this ever happened, but then I know that is wrong and illegal and would not help me. I cannot help but think that I want it all erased, I want all of it to go away, to get away from me, to stop coming back to my life like a chronic infection.

I want it all to go away. Like dirt.

And then I think about bleach. The best part of doing laundry—if there is a best part, more like the least awful part—is finishing a load of whites with more bleach than the instructions call for. I used to love putting the boys' T-shirts, football pants, soccer pants, baseball pants, sheets, pillowcases, towels, and socks all in together—a huge soiled, stained, dirty load—then pouring on the bleach and the strong detergent and knowing all the stains would get carried away. Eradicated. Gone. They ceased to exist. I love bleach. It has the smell of amnesia.

23

SPIN

March 2011

In the same stack of mail today are the MasterCard bill I do not want to open, four separate bills from Rush University Hospital for Colin's concussion treatments, Colin's report card from the high school, and a letter from my former husband with a return address sticker listing his second ex-wife's name (it is crossed out in heavy-handed swipes) and address. I recognize the handwriting: big, loopy, childish. It is just the third letter from him to our house in more than seven years.

Inside is a check for $1,000 on an account in his name listing his mother's address. I wonder which one of these women he is really living with—second ex-wife or mother—and I decide it does not matter. The check is made out to me. It comes with a note dated "26 Feb 11" handwritten in blue ink on a simple white sheet of copy paper—no stationery, no niceties, no formalities. He has taken to the European form of calendar dates.

In the note he says he has read my e-mail about the years of no child support payments. He says he will respond to me soon. In the meantime, he writes that he wishes the boys and me well.

I cashed the check.

I remember back to my twenties when I pictured—literally pictured—our unborn family like a painting, a fertile scene within its finite borders. Clean, sharp angles held a portrait of a family landscape within, a beautiful image that was at once comforting and contained, as well as expansive and limitless. I always felt so lucky to be able to engage in the creation of this scene, this family, these children, this setting, our setting, of our doing, demonstrating the willingness and the desire to be one unit. My illusion was that this picture, this family, would be safe always and nobody would ever want to crawl away or out of the frame, because they knew everything and everywhere else was not able to produce this happy, welcoming warmth. It was home. It was family. Even the sound of those words calms me still.

It continues to baffle me that once inside this picture, not only would someone elect to eject himself from its membership, but that it would never occur to him that such action was wrong. I believed my former husband was still operating under the belief system that his children were accessories. He thought he could cryptically inquire every few years about their well-being but otherwise be completely absent, completely disengaged, withdrawn, invisible. Just blowing smoke into a cavern. That he could go missing with no trace.

But I need the check; Brendan's tuition is due for spring quarter at Ohio State, and Brendan called earlier asking for more swipes on his Buck-ID meal plan. Thirty swipes. Seven dollars each.

Six weeks earlier I sent my former husband an e-mail with one hundred pages of the copied legal documents in .pdf form with the most recent court appearances, motions, and maneuverings. I included a one-page summary of all that he owed in back child support, hundreds of thousands of dollars. I also wrote that I intended to pursue the case with the State's Attorney's office.

I had told myself that for the years he was living in Amsterdam, it was completely pointless to pursue child support. But now that he is living and working in the United States, in Chicago—either at his mother's or his ex-wife's, I will take steps.

"Are you moving to put him in jail?" Weldon asks me every time we speak. He doesn't call him "Dad" or his real name.

I tell him I will pursue it in the next month or so; I need to get through winter quarter, I need to revise my manuscript, I need to get Colin through his treatments, I need to fold the clothes, I need to replace the grout in the bathroom, paint the kitchen cabinets, finally learn how to use the curling iron on my hair, graduate from roller derby class into intermediates, maybe grow my hair longer.

I have had a lifetime quota of legal conflicts and am not eager to go back in the ring. My official stance is that I do not feel engaging in a legal fight to incarcerate their father for nonpayment of support is something that would make me proud. Each one of the boys tells me—often—that is what they want me to do.

"Do it for us, Mom," Brendan says. "You need to show him he cannot just walk away and pretend we do not exist." Usually the conversation ends more colorfully: "I want his ass in jail."

Most days I am trying to reconcile with myself the notion that this fatherlessness my boys live through is not ultimately my fault. I am trying to disassociate from his disconnection, and making the equation of parenting not include him, not even as an asterisk. We are complete as a family without him. We are not a broken home. We are not broken. I am enough. They have other men to love who will fulfill a fatherly role.

I listen to other mothers tell stories of their growing children—happy stories—and I wonder if that can possibly be true all the time. Or if they are delusional or deliberately skipping the less than optimal parts. Does no one else have a flip side to the framed family photographs?

Truth is, it is difficult to be a mother, a parent, even when you have a partner who holds up his half of the house. Truth is, even if you are by yourself, you are never really holding up your house alone.

We have a not-so-old washing machine that may be on its last legs. It is my third washing machine in this house in sixteen years. I know one washing machine is supposed to last that long in total, but in our house they just don't—none of them do, no matter the brand, no matter the type, no matter how much they cost. I do about three full loads of laundry a day when the boys are all home—one full load a day when it is just Colin and me in the house—his workout clothes, towels, my workout clothes.

I am currently in full-blown denial about the washing machine and that it should be replaced. It does not spin. Let me revise that; it does not spin without an intervention. It stops on the dial at the spin cycle. It only took me one or two loads of dripping wet clothes to see the problem. So to dry the clothes past dripping wet, I have to open the top and manually turn the basket with one arm, with the dial set to spin and one finger pressing in the hole where the top should be, so the basket will move at all. It takes three, four, five of my Fred Flintstone–starting-the-car turns to get it moving, then *fwack*, I lift my finger and let the top of the machine come down. I pray the spinning continues and I have tricked the basket into spinning. I watch the hose in the cement tub to be sure water is coming out to prove the spin cycle is working.

Most of the time it does. A few minutes later, when the spin cycle stops on its own, the clothes are dry enough to hang or throw in the dryer (which also could stand to be replaced because it can only take a small towel, some socks, and underwear at one time). No appliance in our home is in peak shape. You would never know, looking at the clean clothes in our closets or on our backs, smelling the clean sheets, admiring the clean guest towels in the bathroom off the kitchen, that the spins are not automatic. I intervene.

I can't change the way it has worked out for my sons. I wish I had chosen better for a husband, I wish that their father had been the man he said he was and the father I imagined he would be, long ago in my twenties when he was young and handsome and full of promises. My sons deserve better.

My close friend Susy recently sent me an e-mail that she was moving out of our neighborhood to be closer to a man she had been dating for a few years since an unpleasant divorce. She had been living in her late mother's condo, and her youngest son was now out of high school and she saw no reason to stay in the same suburb. Her boys were grown. She is thinking she may marry this man. She wrote:

> *Life is good. Money is tight with two in college, but you know that story. Still I am happy. Jim is one reason, but I found that happy point before he came and he just helped move the dial further. I decided to be happy. As simple as that sounds, it made a huge difference in my life and how I filter all that happens.*

I tell my sons all the time that being happy is not the goal of life, it is a by-product of doing what you are here to do, finding your bliss by fulfilling your broader dreams of where you fit in the world. You can be happy eating a cheeseburger. Taking a nap. Watching the Discovery Channel. Life is more than that. There is happy from immediate pleasure, and then there is lifelong happy that sometimes hurts along the way. I am not sure if I am right or not. But I do know this: from now on, I choose happy.

24

IMPERFECT

January 2012

I t's a Friday night in January and I am in a Coralville, Iowa, hotel room, a little weary from the four-hour drive from Chicago west on I-88 and then even farther west on I-80, past texting truck drivers and horizontal snow winds, miles of empty ice-dusted fields, and about a hundred signs for Subway. It's comforting knowing all those Subways all over the country house all the same ingredients—chicken cubes, marinated meatballs, peppers, wheels of tomatoes, lettuce confetti, loaves of Italian herb bread sliced swiftly. There was no need for me to stop at one along the way; I just finished putting six turkey, cheese, and spinach sandwiches I made this morning and about a gallon of Vitaminwater in the small humming refrigerator in room 226 of the Comfort Suites. Colin can eat tomorrow after the weigh-ins for the Iowa City West High School quad against Apple Valley—the top-ranked Minnesota team—Iowa City, and suburban Chicago Marmion Academy high schools.

This is one of my final road trips in nine years of high school wrestling for all three of my sons. I am exhausted, nervous, excited, eager. I want Colin to win; I don't want Colin to get hurt. I want to laugh with the other parents in the stands. I want to just for a handful of hours stop thinking about the rest of my life—the pile of bills, Brendan's dilapidated apartment, Weldon's whereabouts in Spain where he is in graduate school, my students, meetings, seminars, ungraded papers, upcoming court dates, freelance deadlines, the snow piling on my front porch steps, the weight I need to drop from Christmas cheesecake.

On the way here I was listening to a 1970s and 1980s radio station from the Quad Cities that lasted at least one hundred miles of the trip. So between Stevie Nicks, Journey, and Stevie Wonder, I was woozy from a buffet of emotions—scoops of pride, relief, nostalgia, and grief. With a windshield view of gray ice ribbon pavement stretched before me, I started to think of all the miles I have logged as a wrestling mom, some alone, some with Colin or Brendan in the backseat, some with Caryn at the wheel—wrestling moms have as much stamina and vigor as any screaming sports fan I have ever seen on ESPN. Except we never paint our foreheads or bellies.

I have spent probably thousands of hours logged in the stands for what amounts to fourteen years when I count youth wrestling plus high school. I have heard the shrill screech of billions of whistles, sometimes so loud my ears pop and I feel fogged in from the noise, unable to concentrate on any one sound. And every week, every season, some of the same scenes play out, over and over, like renditions of *Cats* or *Rent* in musical theaters in suburban strip malls across America. The only thing I have done more of in my life than watch wrestling is work. And sleep. Yes, sleep comes second.

Tomorrow for most all of the day I will be in another high school gym, this one in Iowa City. Oh yes, I have learned that all high school gyms across America look pretty much alike—sure, they have different school colors and mascots and some stands even have backs to the seats—but once you are sitting in the stands, the view is pretty much the same. The lessons I have learned watching wrestling have been not just about the sport.

I have learned not to look away, to be present or you will miss something. If there are six or eight mats in a gym, all with simultaneous wrestling matches, you could have a piece of lint in your eye or chat with the mother next to you and miss your son's match entirely. You have to pay attention. Listen for his name. Follow him to make sure you know where he will be. Then keep watching. The three two-minute periods feel like an eternity when your son is up against someone who looks like he is made of metal, but you need to concentrate, watch carefully, and pay attention. Life, like a wrestling match, goes by quickly. The clock moves relentlessly forward. Daydream and you will miss the entire reason you are here.

This is not to parrot the cliché many soon-to-be empty-nesters say about childhood flashing past. I do not feel any part of my sons' childhoods went quickly; I do not even feel they all went well. I feel I gave raising my sons all I had, and all my imperfections and impatience came along for the ride. I do feel that now that the boys are twenty-three, twenty-one, and eighteen, their childhoods are pretty much over. That is not to say that I will stop telling them to brush their teeth, be polite, study harder, or call me when they arrive somewhere. That is not to say that I do not worry about what kind of men they will be—are. That is to say that I am pretty much finished with the intense parenting part. And it is humbling to look back.

My sons didn't like me all the time—and yes, as preposterous as it sounds now, I expected that they would. Our house was not always a calm or predictable haven from the rest of the world's injustices and chaos. Sometimes it was downright awful. I yelled. They all yelled. Unspeakable things were said. Apologizes were delivered. I punished. I took cell phones. I confiscated video controllers. I enforced bans. I took the car keys and hid them. Sometimes they couldn't find them. I cried at night. I cried in the car driving to work. I speed-dialed them over and over so they would answer my calls. I waited up. I waited in the car. I waited in the gym. I waited in the doctor's office. I waited in the emergency room. I waited in the front hall, clutching my cell phone, peering down the block, holding my breath at 3 AM, praying to see the headlights of the Nissan Altima before it pulled into the driveway. And then I could breathe.

I complained. Not always, but I complained. When I was tired, when I had eighteen-hour days, when their sweat-soaked workout clothes made the basement smell like a sewer, when the teachers called, when they asked for more money than I had, even though I worked several jobs in addition to teaching just to keep us all afloat. I complained when they swore because they thought I wasn't listening, when they didn't ask how I was. I should not have complained. I am sorry that I could not always see with the perspective I have now that this part is almost done. I should have always been grateful. I am now—mostly—I am now.

Because what happens when you raise children as the only parent with all your vulnerabilities showing like neon on snow—through their heartbreak, your illness, and disappointments—is that you raise them without filters. They yell at you because they can. They tell you their secrets because they want to. They hold your heart, not as hostage, but as willing captive. They don't ask you to go to a tournament because they already know you will. They don't acknowledge your presence sometimes because they know you will still appear no matter what. They have to know you will always do what they need to have done, even if they scream in a teenage hurricane that they hate you.

On any given Saturday, or for that matter Thursday or Friday night, I am quite sure I could have found something else to do other than watch my sons wrestle. Put in a load of laundry. Go grocery shopping. Drink wine. Sleep late. Read a book. Work. Watch one of those housewives of wherever shows. Go on a date with someone who at first seems plausible. Go for a walk. Think. But I chose to be present for them. And I truly have to believe that it mattered.

25

ZERO

February 2012

B ob, my attorney, told me not to bother going to court for the status hearing on the "motion to strike all references to educational expense claims in respondent's motion for sum certain." I had not gone to any of them—and there were more than six—since my former husband first started filing motions to dismiss support in the fall of 2011. There were forever the continuances and the requests for more documentation, a cycle of rhetoric and inaction. He had filed a motion for all documents, photos, tapes, electronic messages, and files bearing my name and the names of my boys. That would literally be hundreds of thousands, possibly millions, of documents. Then it was dismissed.

"I'll let you know," Bob said.

My former husband was attempting to prove he did not owe the seven years of court-ordered back child support or college expenses because he had no money and I didn't need the money. He insisted I had secret accounts for the boys' education, said I was not forthcoming with all my assets. I don't know where or what I was supposed to be hiding, but if I did have any of these hidden accounts, I sure would get better haircuts, and maybe not eat lunch at my desk every day. For sure, I'd have the cleaning lady come more than once every six weeks.

He claimed for himself annual incomes of zero for the past several years and had the tax returns to prove it. Zero. Yes, though he was flying between Amsterdam and Chicago, living, working, eating, he had no income. None. No money for travel, food, shelter. A former litigating attorney for one of the most prestigious firms in the city and editor of the law review at a major Catholic law school, and he made less money than Colin did in a weekend of dog-sitting for the neighbor's two bulldogs. I swallowed a missile of fury.

"What did you eat today?" I wanted to ask. "Berries and leaves?"

But I didn't go to the court appearances, partly because of my teaching schedule at Northwestern and partly because years ago my heart had exterminated him. I had no room left for his chaos. Bob went in my stead. Still, I was curious.

"What does he look like?" I asked Bob.

"Thin. Weird."

I didn't ask what he was wearing, though I did want to know if it was a neatly pressed suit. It didn't really matter. I knew better than to update any of the boys about these latest proceedings, even hint that there were any more. I had learned my lesson. At the close of the summer of 2007, shortly before Weldon left for college, when their father first launched his legal maneuvers to avoid child support, I had made what I thought was a reasonable request at home. I had asked each one of the boys to please be exceptionally cooperative and understanding of my level of stress and to not add to or create any conflict. In other words, let the house just be peaceful.

"Your dad is bringing me to court," I had said to each of them. "I need it to be calm at home."

All I really wanted was for them to put their dirty clothes in the laundry room, maybe empty the dishwasher once in a while, come home when they said they would, or clean up after themselves before I got home from work. I hated leaving a house full of sleeping boy-men, cleaning it all up, working a full day, then coming home to boy-men and some of their boy-men friends on the couch with a mess in every room. Having the house be somewhat neat would help counter my feeling that my life was out of my control. It's funny how their made beds allowed me to feel a semblance of order. Funny how a sink without dirty dishes made me feel as if I had it going on.

"Your dad wants to declare you emancipated and have all child support forgiven, past, present, and future."

I may as well have unpinned a grenade in the living room or set them on fire. Selfish and foolish of me; I know that now. I don't know why I didn't realize how explosive that information was, how painful that was for a son to hear. Of course the boys did not care about my level of stress right then. Of course this was not about me. All they heard and all they felt was that their father wanted to discard them, dissolve all responsibility, be done with his children. Pretend they don't need. Pretend they don't live.

I should never have said a word. My request was absurd, like asking you to please be quiet while I amputate your hand.

What followed were weeks of rigid tension, fights over nothing, raw hurt translated into aggression. Each son was quick to defend or attack. They all fought with me and each other over the smallest indignations—who ate the last piece of chicken, who lost at a video game. And no one made his bed.

Now, after five years of legal annoyances and denial of support, I was having dinner with my friend Michele, who is a divorce judge. I told her how exasperated I was. But she told me I probably should go to the court date in February, to show my former husband I wasn't intimidated. She said I needed to be there to be a real person to the judge, not just a respondent, someone's client, a faceless name in a file. But going would be difficult; I had a class all Tuesday afternoon, a graduate-level editing class with sixteen students ranging from twenty-three to thirty-three years old. One of the students in my class was a younger sister of a student I taught as an undergraduate, another was a man in his thirties who studied at the Sorbonne and came to graduate school after serving in the military for seven years. I wanted to go to class; besides, it is almost impossible to get a stand-in for a four-hour class.

I didn't go to court; it was continued anyway.

■ 26 ■

EMBRACE

February 2012

Three days later Colin was wrestling in individual state sectionals. He needed to be in the top four to qualify for individual state, the opportunity to win a medal, what he had been planning for and working for his entire high school wrestling career. "You are steps away from the top of the mountain," Colin said Coach Powell told all the wrestlers.

I had watched Coach Powell speak to the boys in the lobby of the Holiday Inn in Pontoon Beach, Illinois, the night before the Granite City tournament. All the boys gathered near the pancake machine, toaster, and juice dispenser, some kneeling near a locked refrigerator that held the contents for a free breakfast.

The wrestlers from our team took up almost all of the chairs in the room, but two boys from another team sat at another table tapping on their laptops. They stopped to listen to Coach Powell. The room was silent, each bedraggled son in sweatpants and fleece jacket, his worn wrestling bag at his feet, rapt in attention.

215

"This is about courage and determination," Coach Powell said. They looked at him, silent and believing, like he was Moses.

Ranked eleventh in the state, Colin's record was good, twenty-nine wins, nine losses. I had seen most every one of those matches this year. One very important match I almost missed. It was the time I flew in from San Francisco on the 6 AM flight after co-leading a seminar at Stanford. I landed at O'Hare after noon, raced to the high school, which was twenty minutes from the airport, and had another mom from the team meet me at the front, take my car, and park it in the high school parking lot so I would not miss any of Colin's match. I ran inside the field house to catch Colin one minute into the first period of his match. And I saw him win.

It was like this every weekend, at every dual, every tournament. We were all cheering in the stands, screaming loud, responding with our silly team mantra after each win for each of the wrestlers, "Who let the dogs out?" Then we would all bark.

"You sound crazy, Mom," Colin said.

Colin had never gotten downstate since he was on varsity his sophomore year. He had MRSA after winning regionals that year; he got the severe concussion junior year at the Huskies Tournament the end of January, two weeks before regionals. This was his last chance. As a senior this was the last time he would be able to be as good as his older brother was, as good as everyone believed he could be. He could be a champion, prove to the outside world he was great at this. He could be someone with a state medal, someone who deserved it all, even if his own father never knew, even if his own father would have to read about it online or in the local paper.

Coach Powell and Coach Paul Collins always told Colin he was good enough to be on the medal stand at state. Colin could dominate anyone in the wrestling room near his weight; he had beaten the Wisconsin state champion in January. He had beaten wrestlers with better rankings. All Colin had to do was believe it—go out on the mat confident enough to win.

Weldon had been calling every day from Madrid, where he was getting his master's in contemporary Spanish history. The night before Weldon talked to Colin for more than an hour, telling him how he deserved to win, how he needed to win, how he was a champion.

"It's your circle," he said to Colin. "You don't let anybody take your circle." I could hear Weldon almost shouting over the phone.

Brendan texted Colin from his apartment in Columbus, just a few blocks from the Ohio State University campus, the apartment with rats in the basement and squirrels in the attic. It was the kind of student housing that makes every mother's stomach churn.

"You can do it, Colin," he wrote.

It was snowing in the afternoon and I was worried about how long it would take to get from my campus in Evanston to De La Salle High School at 35th Street and Michigan Avenue on the South Side of Chicago, just about ten miles. Traffic could slow to a near stop on Lake Shore Drive when it snowed. The first matches were at 4:30 PM, so I left my office a little after 3 PM.

Colin had been OK in the morning, a little nervous. He didn't want to talk before he left for school and I left for work. He had to make weight—138 pounds in the newer weight classes set in 2011—so he was irritable. He packed two turkey, spinach, and cheese sandwiches for after the weigh-ins and three bottles of pink Vitaminwater. He would leave on the team bus straight from school.

"What can I do to help you?" I asked Colin.

He shrugged. "Love you, Mom," he said as he shut the back door.

All the other moms from our team were in the stands when I arrived carrying the stuffed Siberian husky we dressed in a singlet and headgear. It's the dog we call "Champ" that Caryn bought in 2009. We take turns waving him above our heads whenever a wrestler on our team wins. Pat, the mother of the heavyweight, starts the cheer. Otherwise, Champ sits in the stands. After the matches for 106, 113, 120, 126, and 132 pounds, Colin was up. Four mats were going at once, so we could get out at a reasonable hour. This was the preliminary round; the champions from regionals had a bye. Colin had come in second at regionals, so he needed to wrestle this one.

His opponent was a wrestler with a record not as strong as Colin's—twenty-four wins, six losses—but Colin looked uncertain. I could see it on his face; sometimes he seemed lost, as if he just woke up from a dream and was surprised to be there. It was a close match, a lot of scrambling, and when the buzzer sounded at the end of the third period, Colin had lost 5–4. After shaking hands with the winner and the other team's coaches, he ran off the mat and disappeared into the back hallways of the school, where another group of mothers was putting up red foil Valentine decorations for the sweetheart dance that night. I knew better than to follow him.

I have learned that my boys are not like me after they suffer a disappointment or a heartbreak. I want to cry, I want someone to listen to me, tell me I am OK, tell me anything I need to hear. But my sons want to be left alone, and they want nothing to do with anyone, least of all me. I have come to accept that and it is OK. Though every part of me wants to talk to him, hug him, soothe him, I know that is not at all what Colin wants or needs.

I knew that he was hard on himself. I knew that Coach Powell was furious at him, not just for losing, but for not letting himself win. Powell was not going to let Colin get away with losing, not believing in himself. Powell was going to yell at him good. He was going to make him cry.

But the reality is that half of the wrestlers in every equation are losers. Not good odds when you think about it. I think of the sport and the years of my boys on the mat, and I remember the victories, the rumbling din of clapping, shouting, and hugging the other moms. But for each match, one of those two boys slinks away, head lowered, shamed, beaten. Sometimes the loser blames the ref, the call, a poked eye, a wrenched shoulder, a twisted ankle, but I know, really know, each wrestler blames himself. It is hard to watch that torment in anyone's son. It is almost unbearable to watch in your own.

You sit in the stands so long for so many Saturdays over so many years that you see just how much each win or loss means to these young men and you see how some parents handle it well and some parents, well, some parents you want to just vanish. Some parents boo the boys and the refs. Today two fathers got in a shouting match in one corner of the gym, where more than a thousand parents and athletes pace, gaze, or fume. Some parents make snide comments about your son or your team just loud enough so you can hear them. Some of the mothers cry in the stands while friends or sisters or mothers console. Some fathers storm off enraged. The whole day is loud, uncomfortable, and confrontational as the whistles bounce off the tiled gym walls and the teenagers step on your coat or your shoes climbing over you to get to the concession stand, bringing back plastic boats of orange cheese they will likely spill on your back.

What you want to say is, "It's just wrestling," but you know it isn't. It's like telling me, "It's just a book" or "It's just a class," but it is more than that. It is a metaphor for your identity, your worth, your intention, your dreams. It is a measure of how far you have come, how big you have dreamed, how far you have dared to go. It means everything. It is more than just high school wrestling, even if you don't want it to be.

Weldon called four times on my cell phone, but I didn't hear it ring in the din of the high school gym. Brendan texted. I texted him back. I e-mailed Weldon and texted him that Colin lost. I knew he would call later.

Going into individual state finals, our team was first in the state for this year; we won our conference and dominated every tournament, sometimes winning by one hundred team points or more. Coach Powell was looking healthy for the most part, not as thin as he was in 2009, but thicker, more like himself. He got a new haircut and grew his beard, as he did every year leading up to state. He acted as if he felt OK, though sometimes he limped when he stood up from the stands or walked awkwardly when he left the chair at the side of the mat at the end of a match. He never complained. If you asked, sometimes he just smiled.

"I'm OK, my numbers are down," he would say. Then he would change the subject.

His father, Bud, talked about going on vacation for a week with his wife, his son, and his son's wife in St. Lucia, after team state.

"He's depleted," he said.

But Coach Powell had been able to take the seniors on the trip last summer to Angel's Landing in Zion National Park. They hiked for two days in Bryce Canyon National Park. One photo from the trip shows all the boys with their shirts off on a mesa—plus a shirtless Coach Powell beaming alongside Coach Collins and Coach Boyd. Colin has the framed photo in his room on the nightstand next to his bed; all the seniors had the same framed photo. Coach Powell gave it to each senior on senior night at the high school.

The rest of the night there were plenty of wins for our team. Nine of the boys held out hopes for state; they would be the state qualifiers Colin planned to be.

The next morning was a chance for wrestle-backs, the consolation round; Colin could still make it to state if he won three matches today.

I got to the gym with Caryn about 9:30 AM. Wrestling started at 10 AM and my brother Paul showed up shortly after that, asking where the coffee was. With four matches concurrently, it all moved pretty quickly. Colin's youth football coach, Tim O'Dell, showed up to watch Colin. He had come to the high school a handful of times this season with his son Tommy to cheer Colin on.

Colin was up against a wrestler from a school outside our conference who had a 27–12 record. He had never wrestled him before so I didn't know what to expect. From the first whistle, Colin dominated, and he won 8–5. Coach Powell was pleased, handed him his shorts and sweatshirt after the match, and went to the side with him to go over some moves. Colin was still in it. He could still go to state.

Between matches, I went over to Colin in the stands and kissed him on the top of his head. He let me.

"Thanks, Mom," he said.

The next match would be easy for Colin, up against a wrestler with a 19–3 record, someone who Colin seemed to dominate early on. Paul and I were crouched on the sidelines, cheering.

"You got this, Colin," Paul screamed.

It looked in the first period like Colin would win, and then all of a sudden it was over. He was pinned. And Colin lost his chance for individual state.

I didn't see Colin for at least an hour; I am not sure where he went. I waited in the stands and knew he would come back when he was ready. Paul said he went to look for him and found him sitting by himself, silent, distraught. Paul hugged him and told him he had a great season and that winning did not matter as much as giving it your all. He had a good season. He could be proud.

Later in the afternoon, before the break in sessions, I saw Coach Powell approach Colin and hug him, another long embrace. From where I sat in the stands across the gym, it was a sight that I pray will stay with me for years.

You don't have to win to be loved.

Monday shortly after noon, following a two-hour undergraduate Magazine Storytelling class, I was in my office on a conference call, listening to about a dozen people speak back and forth, occasionally inserting a question or responding. My cell phone vibrated on my desk and I could see it was Coach Powell. I hung up on the conference call. I needed to take this.

"How is Colin?" Coach Powell's voice was raspy, deeper than usual.

"Devastated, but OK. He'll be OK."

"Colin could have won, he beat one of those kids twice already," he said. "But what's important is that he got the lessons from wrestling that he needed. In the end it doesn't matter how you did in high school wrestling, nobody cares. It matters what kind of man you are, and Colin is a good man."

I started to cry. Noon on a Monday morning in my office overlooking south campus.

"I'll talk to him," he said.

I started to babble about how much I appreciated Coach Powell and what he has done for my boys, how much I wanted Colin to have that feeling of winning, having his hand raised in the air in an assembly hall of screaming fans. I said I could not have raised these boys without his influence, that I was grateful for all his efforts.

"He can have that feeling later in life," Powell said. And, he reminded me, although Colin had lost his shot at individual state, he would still be able to wrestle at team state if the Huskies qualified. He paused. "Part of this is about you. You let all your boys go into this sport and you let them be who they are."

Maybe it is because I am a writer, but sometimes I see my life played out in scenes. *I could write this that way,* I think as someone is laughing or walking away. This was a scene with the music swelling up, the teary ending. The not-so-happy ending, but the one where you know in your bones it will all be OK. It's the ending where the hero reveals himself, the villain recedes, and you know the lessons have been learned. But then I knew it wasn't really an ending at all.

We had to beat the Hinsdale Central team to qualify for team state. It was set for Tuesday, February 21, at 6 PM, barely enough time for me to drive there after my graduate editing class ended at 5 PM. So I let my students work on their captions assignments and e-mail them to me. I was in the car by 4:40 PM.

Once at the field house, the atmosphere was loud and anxious. Parents of wrestlers who graduated four or even five years ago showed up and took their places in the stands. Peter Lovaas, who wrestled with Weldon and graduated in 2007, climbed up to a seat next to his father. The grandfather from Wisconsin who drives to see more than half of our matches, whose own son wrestled in the 1960s, was there in the stands taking notes and wearing his HUSKIES WRESTLING FAMILY T-shirt.

I took out my camera. The boys from the team came running down from the wrestling room, and after they were introduced by weight—along with the opposing team—the captains went to the center of the mat to shake hands. I started taking pictures. I caught Coach Powell's eye as he looked at me in the stands.

"This is the last one," he mouthed.

"I know," I said and laughed.

The dual began at 182 pounds and the team won the first three matches handily—182, 195, 220. Colin would wrestle at 145 pounds; Powell had worked out the lineup to maximize effectiveness. He had talked to the boys before the match—as he always did—and they each looked pumped, charged, and electrified, ready to take on the world for six minutes. Before he went out, Coach Powell hugged Colin for what looked like a long time but was probably only a minute or so.

Colin burst onto the mat and then dominated the entire match. He won 12–3. I screamed so loud I should have been embarrassed, but I wasn't. Colin had come back, believed in himself again, pushed himself as hard as he could.

He would prepare to wrestle at team state in Bloomington, Illinois, his last year, Powell's last year. And though they came home from Bloomington after a hard-fought day—winning first against Harlem and later against Barrington—they lost in the final round to the Sandburg team and took the second-place trophy.

It didn't seem like it that night to Colin or to any of the wrestlers on the team, not even the coaches, but it was good enough. For me, it was enough.

When Weldon was born, I told the nurses at Medical City in Dallas that he would be a senator or author as the owner of such a regal name. This was not the moniker of someone to be taken lightly; this was someone destined for greatness, someone I wanted the world to know. Before he spoke coherent words, I listened intently to his babbling, waiting for the first sign that he understood me and that I understood him. I couldn't wait for him to talk. So many millions of words exchanged since then—some harsh, some tender, many only I would hear—and now that he is twenty-six, I can't wait to hear what he has to say when he calls. When he was earning his master's degree in Madrid and traveling on weekends, he would call from Portugal, Italy, Morocco, or wherever he was on an adventure. And it was thrilling.

I was the kind of mother who pictured my children as adults—
even as infants when I was struggling to maneuver them into their
down-softened, pale-blue snowsuits, their arms and legs flailing, help-
less until I lifted them up like pliable gingerbread men. I was never
the kind of parent who wanted them to stay small, not because it
was so hard, but because I thought it would be so glorious to know
them, well, as people. Full-grown adults.

Yes, I have the scary movies playing in my head when something
goes wrong and I imagine the worst. But most of the time, when I
saw them in the future I saw their greatness years ahead as if looking
into a snow globe—a scene hazy and distorted. I saw them for who
they could be—grown men with broad shoulders and wide smiles—
and I saw myself in the audience at their graduations, their speeches,
their award acceptances, their medal ceremonies, their grand public
gestures. This is the good side of mother vision.

You teach your children to walk, knowing they will eventually
walk away.

You hope that your children know you never will.

27

STARS

May 2012

"Mom, it's my last day of high school," Colin shouted, in his boxers dashing from his room into the bathroom—the one he shares with his brothers when they are at home. It's the bathroom I dare not use, with splashed minty toothpaste all over the mirror, the towels he uses once and drops, the razor and shaving cream he can never manage to put away in the cabinet.

"I'm almost not in high school anymore."

I was aware of the milestone, the way you are aware of a due date when you are pregnant or an anniversary date that ends in 0, a court date on the books for months, or a keynote speech on the calendar months away. I designed an invitation for his graduation party with a photo of Colin and his brothers taken more than ten years ago. In the photo Colin is sandwiched by Brendan and Weldon, who are squeezing him playfully. He looks exasperated, pleading.

The invite went to family members, coaches, wrestling families, and everyone else I knew who adored Colin, a total of more than one hundred people. The moms who knew him since his blond hair stood straight up—earning him the nickname Woodstock, as in Snoopy's bird friend—the teachers who told him they would like a son just like him, the other dads who loved him as if he was their own. The party would be the week after his graduation, and I had already ordered the tent. I love the crisp white tent with the metal frame and the teapot dome—it costs more than it should, but I only have these parties every four years or so. I would make pork tenderloin sandwiches and fresh mozzarella pizzas on naan bread, order the chicken. Colin wanted mashed potatoes, though I steered him to potato salad. Coleslaw doesn't ever move as fast as you would hope; I would make a tossed salad with cherry tomatoes, sliced cucumbers, maybe croutons.

"Let me take a picture before you go."

I had already been up for an hour, made coffee, oatmeal for me, peanut butter on toast with fresh blackberries for Colin, and lunch for both of us. I put the lunches in separate plastic bags with an apple and orange in each, plus a granola bar for him. I had made my bed, thrown in a load of laundry—we can't expect to have enough hot water to take hot showers and do laundry at night—and read the front section of the paper, plus the horoscopes in the back. Bad habit, I admit. Mine read: "concern about finances, social gatherings with friends, stay calm when considering the future." Anybody could write those. Anything could happen.

I was dressed for work, just putting my contacts in and watching a few minutes of *Good Morning America* before deciding whether I wanted to wear the great-looking shoes that hurt or the ones I could walk and stand in all day.

I'll be standing up teaching most of the day. Not-so-cute shoes.

Colin wore his orange polo shirt, dress pants, and shoes. He stood about six feet, posing in the kitchen by the microwave as I snapped his picture; I took photos of the boys on first and last days of school from kindergarten through high school, a practice they mostly did not appreciate. Sometimes they stood by the front door with fresh backpacks, for years and years all of them inches to a foot shorter than me, pushing each other, wrangling for the front row. New shoes, new shirts, new haircuts. Now, all of them over six feet tall.

He kissed me good-bye, "Love you, Mom," and forgot to take out the garbage bag or the recycling.

I didn't tell him. I didn't tell Brendan or Weldon either. I didn't say that the previous day I had been in court and had seen their father—for the first time in years, the first time since his own father's funeral. There was no point in telling the boys; it only made them furious. Weldon would only say that I should move to put him in jail for delinquency on child support. Seven years of delinquency, going on eight. No, I said nothing, it could only be hurtful. Who needs to know his father is still fighting to erase his obligations to him? It had been many years since their father saw the boys or communicated to them. Silence. He had missed so much. He had denied them so long.

Fifth grade—Colin was in fifth grade the last time their father had paid any support. There had been a lot of turkey sandwiches since then, a lot of wrestling matches, a bin of wrestling medals.

I once again donned a medal of my own the previous day when I prepared to see my former husband. My father's gold medal hangs on a heavy gold chain that falls to the middle of my chest. On one side of the cracker-sized disc is an image of Mary holding Jesus as an infant. She has a halo, a crown really, and the medal is framed in elaborate filigree. On the flipside of the medal in capital letters is engraved: WM G WELDON, and underneath his name is his social security number. It is the medal he wore every day as a solider in World War II. He told me once it is what kept him alive; he believed the talisman saved him. When he died my sisters gave it to me.

When my father died in January 1988, none of my boys were born; Weldon arrived in October of that year. None of the boys knew their grandfather, Papa Bill, though many remark that Brendan resembles him—his oval, handsome face and dimpled chin. Each one of the boys has his kindness.

My brother Paul lent Colin Papa Bill's cufflinks to wear to his graduation later in June.

"This is the first thing I ever had of his," Colin said and gave Paul a bear hug.

I don't wear my father's medal often; I only wear it when I need his strength—important speeches, meetings, and a court date like today. I hadn't gone to the half dozen other appearances in the past six months, of him presenting motions and interrogatories about my finances, claiming that although he owes hundreds of thousands of dollars in unpaid child support and college expenses, I do not need financial help. I imagine he expected child support to be dismissed as quickly as his law loans were after he filed bankruptcy.

"He can't do that," friends would say to me.

Yes, he can.

It was time to go to court and at least be the face of the respondent. I dreaded the idea of reliving it all again, of having to face the person who hurt my sons. I did not have a class on Thursday morning at Northwestern; I could go to court. I needed to go, in spite of the stress-induced nausea, in spite of the trembling I could not control in my hands. Benign familial tremor: a doctor diagnosed it years ago when I was married to him. Your body remembers.

A plain black skirt, plain black jacket, simple white blouse. Pumps with low heels, we would walk to the courthouse from my sister Madeleine's new law office near the federal building. Drew, an attorney in her firm, was now handling the case since I couldn't afford an attorney. Madeleine was allowing Drew to do this for free. It cost my former husband nothing to keep filing motions because he is an attorney. So he kept filing.

I wanted my mother with me. She would know what to say. She would hold her head high—even from a wheelchair. But she has been gone a decade; I wore her gold bracelet, the one that has three rows of beads and clasps with a click. There. I am safe now. My father's medal, my mother's bracelet, both my parents are with me.

I talk to my late parents often; I am not sure it is praying really, although sometimes I cry at night, "Please, Mom, help me," and I pause and wait for some kind of response, relief, respite. And I search my heart and memory for what she would do. I squint my lids shut tighter and try to see if I can see her in my mind's eye, but I can't. I try to channel her bravado and her wit, think of how she would respond, think of how she would end a conversation with a remark so insightful it was stunning. Think of how she would soothe me when bullies chased me home in fourth grade. "It's just a dog barking, Mich. Makes no more sense than a dog barking, and no need to cry over a barking dog." If she knew that my former husband had nothing to do with her grandsons, she would be furious. She would call up his mother and she would give her a piece of her mind. Oh yes, she would.

"Behave with the good sense your parents gave you," she said to my former husband once after our divorce when he came to pick up the boys for a visitation. He looked at the floor. But it never changed.

My sisters and I have this thing; I don't know if it really is anthropomorphism, but I'll just say it: My mother is a butterfly, and lately my father is a cardinal. Every spring and summer butterflies flock to my back porch; one usually lands on the glass table when the boys and I eat dinner outside. One will land on a book I am reading in the sun. They will flit in stops and starts on the lilac bushes, the verbena, the hibiscus, the scented geraniums my friend Katherine told me to buy. Many spring and summer mornings a bright red cardinal sits alone on the telephone wire stretched across my backyard or on the basketball rim, of all places. Just sits. For several minutes. Most every day.

"Hi, Dad," I say. And I don't care who hears me.

The benches in Judge Naomi Schuster's courtroom are filling up; we are there only a few minutes before 10 AM. I glance around the room; he is not here. A thirty-ish woman in a red sweater has a lip ring, nose ring, and a diamond piercing in the area between her mouth and nose. I think that would hurt. A woman to my right is chewing gum loudly and holding a stack of papers. Drew motions me to sit down in the front row and she sits to my right. Six rows are filling with men and women—all with blank faces, staring ahead.

A woman is standing before the judge with an attorney to her left. She is dressed in a postal uniform.

"All I know is he lives in Cleveland," she tells the judge.

"How long has he lived in Cleveland?"

"A couple of years," she said.

She tells the judge she has not received support for her three children. I cross my legs and shift in my seat. Another couple approaches the judge's bench when their names are called.

"Two of the children are emancipated," an attorney says.

"I agree to support my youngest child," the man says sheepishly.

The judge assigns terms to the payment.

My former husband rushes in. I see him out of the corner of my eye and do not move to face him; I sense him. He sees Drew and does a double take when he sees me. I do not look up, I do not make eye contact. But I can see him. His hair is long, well below his collar, and he is wearing a trench coat, a black suit, a white shirt, nice shoes, a tie. He sits next to Drew. My chest starts to tighten.

He sits on the end of the row; Drew is between us. I try not to move, to act flustered, but my body is tightening. I am aware of him in my skin the way an animal is aware of a possible predator. He does not sit still. I see him bend down, his upper body flush to his legs, a sort of yoga pose, as if he is stretching, gathering himself. It is so odd I nudge Drew with my elbow. Drew looks ahead. He sits up straight and does it again suddenly; a bending bow, his chest touching his legs as he sits, his hands touching the floor.

At least ten more names are called. It is nearly 11 AM. His name is called—he is bringing forth the motions and I am the respondent—and I approach the bench and stand near my former husband for the first time in many years. I say nothing. Drew advised me to say nothing.

Spots start swirling in front of me, as if I am going to faint; an expanding wallpaper of stars unfolds in front of my eyes. I cannot possibly fall down. Not now. Not here. My chest and head are so hot I feel incinerated. *Breathe through your mouth. Calm down. Don't speak.* Drew told me not to speak.

Drew answers the judge's questions. The judge never looks at me.

"Your honor, I was assured when the boys were born, that college would be paid for," my former husband says.

"By whom?" my attorney asks.

"By her family," he responds.

My father died before my sons were born. My mother died in 2002.

Back and forth, back and forth, the pulse in my ears is nearly deafening and my breath is heaving and loud. I try to relax. I can't. Drew requests he supply the last two years of income tax statements. Even though he has claimed on the statements that he still lives in the Netherlands, he has filed US tax returns with an income claim of zero. $0. The law review editor at a top private university. Former litigating attorney at a top firm. $0.

In my head I am screaming. *How do you live on zero income? How do you eat? How are you wearing a new suit?*

And then it's over. I have to come back in twenty-one days. More answers to his questions. And then a hearing. And then a trial. I cannot have a trial. I do not want to spend any more time responding to him. I only want him to do what is right. For his sons. I go back to the bench and pick up my briefcase and raincoat and leave the courtroom, but not before I see my former husband mouth the words, "I would like to speak to Michele."

Drew asks me in the hallway and I say yes.

"Michele, I want to be clear there are two separate issues: My insolvency is one issue. My gratitude for you paying for the boys' college is another. I am grateful for all you have done." He looks at me. I draw in a deep breath.

I have practiced this, rehearsed this soliloquy in my head ten thousand times. In the car, in the shower. When he misses another Christmas. When I see Colin cry when he says that his own father does not love him. When Brendan is enraged. When Weldon chides me for not putting his father in jail. I rear up and look him in the eye.

Compliment, acknowledge him. I learned this from writing opinion pieces for newspapers, magazines, CNN, from my training I do for The OpEd Project. *Validate the other side.* It keeps the crazy commenters at bay on blog posts, sometimes. At least it does not immediately alienate them. *He loves a compliment. I am ready.*

"You are an intelligent, resourceful, innovative, talented man." And now I come in closer. "And you chose this. Shame on you. You chose to abandon your sons. You choose to have nothing to do with them, not for years."

His face is blank; he does not look surprised, he does not react. He looks at me with all the emotion and involvement of someone staring at a train schedule posted on the wall of Union Station. I search his face for any reaction, I search his face to elicit any recollection in me of a man who is a father, of the man I married twenty-six years earlier. Of the man I divorced sixteen years earlier. Of the man who hurt my sons. I feel this trembling rage simmering inside me. Here is the man whom I believe chose to hurt my boys.

"You have missed it all. The graduations, the hospitalizations, the laughs, the breakups, the awards, the jobs, the flu. It is not just the money, though that has made their lives lean. You have changed who they are."

I feel tears coming into my throat. But I won't let them. I clear my throat. Because this is it. And I tell him why it matters.

"They are sons with a father who does not care at all what they do or who they are. And they are wonderful. Weldon is in graduate school in Spain. Brendan is smart and funny and doing well, finishing his third year at Ohio State. Colin just won this big award—the spirit of the team—in wrestling at Oak Park High. And he is going to the University of Iowa. You don't even know them. You missed it all. Shame on you."

I am not done, but I take a breath. He fills in the pause in a low voice.

"They have not responded to my communication," he says crisply.

But he has told a lie and I will not let it pass.

"You have not communicated to them in any way for five years. Five years. Not one thing. Not a phone call. Not a letter. Not an e-mail. Not on Christmas, not on a birthday. Not any support. They could have used the money. Their lives would have been OK, not so much struggle. But shame on you for the choice you made to have nothing to do with your sons. Snakes know better. They stay with their eggs. You abandoned your own sons."

"I don't have their addresses," he answers.

"We have lived in the same house for sixteen years. And if you write to them, you better goddamn beg for forgiveness. The first three words of anything you write to them better be, 'I am sorry.'"

He starts to say something, then stops, closes his lips. He turns and walks away. My hands are shaking, sweat is pouring down my back. I stood up to the bogeyman. But I don't feel better.

Drew puts her arm around my shoulders. We wait a few minutes and take the elevator to the first floor, past the security checks. Outside it is raining hard, the sidewalks are slick. I press my umbrella open and walk to the garage.

28

FINAL

December 2012

Avoiding a full hearing and without going to trial, we settled. The judge ordered my former husband to give me a cashier's check for $30,000 in accordance with the Joint Settlement Agreement and Release. After two years of court appearances trying to have him pay any of eight years of child support and educational costs, he signed an agreement that with this payment of less than 10 percent of what he owed, he would stop all legal claims against me. And I would in turn relinquish all claims against him for financial support or any kind of support for all three of the boys.

We were done.

In consideration of payment as set forth herein, Weldon hereby completely releases and forever discharges X from any and all child support claims, demands, obligations, actions, causes of action, rights, damages, costs, losses of service, expenses and compensation of any nature whatsoever, included but not limited to alimony, child support, education expense, medical expense or any right pursuant to this divorce decree under Illinois law.

I didn't go to court on December 5; funny, it was my half birthday and my best friend Dana's birthday. Since we were roommates in our freshman year in the Northwestern University Apartments, room 203, on Orrington Avenue, we celebrated our half birthdays in person or by phone. Over thirty-seven years, our twice-annual birthday and half-birthday talks shifted from boyfriends to husbands to ex-husband to should-be ex-husband back to boyfriends to sons.

I had a class that morning and signed off on the agreement by fax to my attorney. I had to make corrections in it; under "Recitals" he had our wedding date wrong, listing it as April 23, 1986, not August. He also wrote that Colin attended Iowa State University. He spelled Brendan's name wrong—with an *o*.

Apparently the appearance in court was uneventful. My former husband handed the check to the judge, who handed it to my attorney. I e-mailed my sister to see if it had gone OK. Later that evening, Madeleine called and said she had a bottle of champagne and wanted me to come over to celebrate the end of this chapter. It had been eighteen years of legal wranglings for a nine-year marriage. Terrible odds of 2:1.

I don't like champagne—it gives me a headache. But I understand its significance. I had a glass.

It's hard to describe how I felt, but mostly I felt relief. Definitely I was incredulous, because it had been almost all of Colin's lifetime that I had been reacting to their father's behaviors. This new state of release had the same surreal fog around it as if I was finding out something all along I believed to be true is now rendered false. The world really is flat! Not a good surprise, but a feeling that you were duped.

I have read that long-term stress deleteriously affects your health and physically changes your brain; specifically your hippocampus. When people say something is a load off their minds, it literally is like that. Your mind is released of a burden, a weight, like lifting a dumbbell off your forehead—the headache is gone. You feel your mind open up, like a black-out window shade lifted in a dark room that had closed up for years. With the shade newly open, you see for the first time it is midday, the sun is bright, and you can breathe.

I felt as though for the past sixteen years since I was divorced, there had been an uncomfortable presence in my life, no matter how much I tried to ignore it, compartmentalize it, pretend it wasn't there. In the past few years, it had been monthly if not weekly appearances in courts, and responses for requests for documents. I worried what he may do next. I worried how whatever he did may hurt the boys—again, more, still, forever. I no longer looked for him lurking in places, but I never felt free of him. Now I do.

I do feel as if I do not have to be afraid anymore—of him and his legal machinations, denials, and unpredictable swipes. And that notion is liberating. I sense a literal lightening, as if my brain and my life are being cleared of debris, making clean a space for new ideas, new adventures, new thoughts, new loves. The past vacuumed away. A clean slate.

With the money from their father, I paid Weldon's second semester tuition at Universidad de Complutense. I paid Brendan's final tuition as a senior at Ohio State. I paid Colin's second semester freshman year tuition at University of Iowa. I paid the electricity, water, gas, and cell phone bills. I let Brendan get a new iPhone. I paid off the $1,100 plane ticket from Madrid for Weldon to come home for Christmas. I paid off the Best Buy credit card for the refrigerator I had to buy last summer when the old one just stopped working. I still have not had the water line connected for the ice maker; the installer wanted $150 for that convenience. I figured some time the boys or a friend of theirs could hook up the water line.

In the meantime, it is not hardship to buy a ten-pound bag for less than two dollars at the grocery store every week. I paid off my MasterCard bill and did some Christmas shopping. I hosted Christmas Eve for my family, twenty-five for dinner. Brendan helped me marinate the salmon and beef filets, roast the potatoes with garlic, olive oil, and sea salt; I splurged. Then all the money from him was gone.

Three weeks later I took my last dose of Femara. I had been on the cancer medication for five years, after the breast cancer surgery and the tamoxifen, and the surgery to remove my ovaries after suspecting I had ovarian cancer but did not. I was considered cured of cancer. I was free. When I told Weldon, he sent me flowers—dozens of alstroemeria in shades of pink, deep red, yellow, and white. There were so many, I put them in four vases so I could have them in different rooms of the house.

It's two clothespins and an egg carton filled with a scrap of folded blue cloth masquerading as Joseph, Mary, and baby Jesus in a manger. The clothespins are Mary and Jesus, respectively; Mary in a mouse-size swath of pale-yellow cotton the color of lemonade, Joseph in striped cloth. Bits of fabric are glued on their heads, their faces inked in marker. Jesus is lying in a torn piece of gray cardboard egg carton—the manger is the spot for a single egg. A square of fabric is folded around a half popsicle stick with a smaller face; Jesus's face. The Savior of the World is propped on top of shredded, crinkled brown strips of paper, the kind they use in fancy wrapping, that usually arrive in gold, silver, or bright colors like pink or blue.

Colin made it fifteen years ago when he was three and in the afternoon session of First United Nursery School, the preschool all three of my boys attended, the one by the public library and the one where they hold graduations every May in the basement and many of the mothers cry.

On the living room Christmas tree—a fake tree with lights attached ("I am so surprised you do not have a real one," my friend Lisa announced) are a dozen rolls of gold wire-rimmed ribbon cascading from bottom to top, where a wire angel the size of my hand grips the tallest fake branch for dear life. I love a real tree—the way it smells, the way the branches spread and droop over the weeks, the daily watering you must do before the sap seals the fresh cut and the needles become so brittle they hurt as you kneel down to put one more present under the tree. But we can't have one.

I always had fresh trees in the apartments I lived in by myself, on Fullerton Avenue then Wrightwood Avenue then Cedar Street in Chicago; Gaston and then Oram Street in Dallas when I was mar ried; Lake Shore Drive in Long Beach, Indiana; White Oak Drive in South Bend; Linden Avenue in Oak Park. And now, in the red brick River Forest house with my boys, for our seventeenth Christmas here, we have a fake tree.

"Do you have a real Christmas tree?" the ear, nose, and throat doctor on North Avenue asked as she peered into Weldon's nostrils. He was five years old.

It was three days before Christmas, Brendan was just two, and I was a few weeks away from delivering Colin.

"Yes," I replied dutifully, struggling to contain Brendan in my minimized lap.

"You have to get rid of it as soon as you can. He is highly allergic."

"Really? Before Christmas?" I was thirty-eight weeks pregnant and so pleased that I had managed to decorate the house at all. Now I had to take it down.

"Yes, he can barely breathe from it. Take it down today."

So I did. And I didn't put up a replacement but promised the boys Santa would place the presents in the spot where the tree had been. We would have a sign indicating as much in case he couldn't figure it out. Neither boy argued. We left out cookies on a plate for Santa and carrots for the reindeer. You can't ignore the reindeer; after all, they do most of the work, and stay out in the cold the whole time.

I was married then, but I don't recall my husband helping with the tree—putting it up or dismantling it, or even hauling it to the street. I remember returning from the doctor and dutifully undressing the tree and putting the decorations in plastic bins, and then dragging the tree out onto the front porch, no doubt causing the neighbors to wonder if we had our calendar skewed. I used to worry about what the neighbors thought—Lou and Rosalie to the south especially. Lou was a kind old man with soft blue eyes who pulled weeds in his backyard in his worn pajamas; his wife was in a wheelchair the last few years of her life. Before that she was a volunteer at the Trailside Museum, where they had raccoons and possums in cages. That always seemed odd to me; all I needed to do was walk past the garbage cans late at night to see the same animals. Lou still sends me Christmas cards. There was the hostile old woman—French—to the north who put up a six-inch-high plastic fence between our front yards because she said I pushed the mower too far outside the lot line and mistakenly cut the grass on her property.

A single woman lived across the street with two young children; I never quite understood who the father was or if she received sperm donations—that was the rumor on the block. I didn't care, it was none of my business, and with all I was going through at the time, using a sperm donor seemed a smart move on her part. I waved to her when I took the boys for walks in the stroller or shoveled the front walk in the snow. The Dohertys lived across the street a few doors to the south with their triplets and older daughter who was Weldon's age—they used to play together on our swing set in the backyard.

I decorated the outside of the house with fresh garland, the inside of the house, the bathrooms, the kitchen, the den, every room in the house to pretend it was happy. It didn't really work.

The only decorations I put on the tree *this* year are ones the boys have made—Weldon's is a triangle-shaped tree with multicolored random puzzle pieces glued to it from at least fifteen years ago. Brendan's is a photo of himself as a third grader glued to a circle of bark and sprinkled with glitter. Colin's is a green paper Christmas tree with colored cotton balls attached with glue.

It will be the ninth Christmas since their father has disappeared from their lives completely. They are not small; they are twenty-four, twenty-one, and eighteen, and they do not believe in Santa Claus. But they do believe in fathers, even if it is a notion afforded only other families, even if they do not believe in their own.

The fatherless space is a hole grand and vacuous and painful, even if only Colin says so. Weldon will dismiss it and Brendan will say his father never really cared about him. I talk to the boys about Barack Obama and tell them to look at what he has done with his life; I throw in Bill Clinton for good measure. Neither had a father growing up. I talk about all the love they do have, about how their father's deliberate absence is about him, not them.

Sometimes I feel as if I am just mouthing words that make no sound as they leave my lips, that they are mere abstract distractions of syllables—sparks of smoke in the face of such gaping wounds. I cannot fix this. I have never been able to fix it, make up for it. I never will. But then I tell myself nothing stays broken forever if you don't want it to—not a life, not a career, not a relationship, not a body, not a family, not a home, not a heart. You can choose to leave behind and escape from the events that led to this aftermath, this space that can be rebuilt and renewed. You can stay forever and try to transform it. You can find what makes you happy in what you do with your days and your mind and hope that it matters, that it creates a space in the world that for someone is edifying. And for you it is uplifting. That's what I chose and I do not think I was wrong in doing so, in spending my life this way, as their mother first. And last.

AFTERWORD

October 2014

As I was making my way to the gate at Washington, DC's, Reagan airport, I got a text from Brendan asking when I would be home. "Don't worry, I cleaned up the house," he wrote.

I had only been gone for thirty-six hours for a seminar I was co-leading for The OpEd Project. How bad could our house be? He was living at home in what we call the man cave in the basement, saving money to move to an apartment.

Minutes later my cell phone rings and it is Weldon asking how I am. I tell him I am trying to get through the TSA security check; he wants to tell me about his day at work in Chicago.

When I sit at the gate, Colin e-mails me from University of Iowa to ask if I can go over his resume because he has a career fair the next morning. I open the document on my phone. I respond to him that he needs to take out the comment that his boss told him he did a "kick-ass" job. He says he will.

And then he writes, "I love you from here to the garage."

That's what he said to me when he was about five or six. I would tell the boys at bedtime that I loved them from here to the moon,

Venus, or Mars. And Colin proclaimed his love for me was from here in his bedroom to the garage, a huge expanse of about one hundred feet. I know what he meant.

There is an inherent contradiction in the proposition of a woman raising men. It is not a sexist thing to say, it is not about culture, it is about otherness. The difference between us can be fraught with peril—the disconnect between what they know and experience and what I project. My sons are mine, but they are not like me.

My boys love risk and daring; I do not even like Ferris wheels. They are quick to react, impulsive. I try to think everything through, weigh every angle, and mostly I err on the side of caution. A quarter of a century into this lab experiment, I can definitively say that the concept of otherness in a relationship doesn't mean you cannot be close. But the differences play out daily.

Anyone who claims there is no inherent opposition in action, attitude, or life approach for mothers and sons simply has not had an experience with sons like mine. Much of the time they believe I am completely wrong. Occasionally they will concede, but not without a volley.

As a parent, mother or father to son or daughter, every day you know there is possibility for delinquency, failure, haphazard mistakes, indelible marks, any and all horrors that become evident only when you are already in so deep you have to be extricated. You fear for your kids. You fear mistakes and missteps that change who they are and that make the future evaporate before it starts.

The examples are there every day for you to read about in the local newspaper, or hear about in the worried phone calls you get from other mothers you've known for years. Bad stuff, really bad stuff can happen to a son or daughter—drugs, alcohol, arrests, violence, burglary, assault, shoplifting, school expulsion, unplanned pregnancy, all of it, any of it. A few almost die from drugs and are forever in rehab. Or they sustain a limp from being in a drug coma curled in a ball in the backseat of a friend's car for two days. And you know, just know, there but for the grace of God, go my children.

So as a single mother, the only parent charged with these sons, the only one of their parents paying attention, it feels miraculous when something awful doesn't go down, like you are watching a tornado whip through your neighborhood from the safety of the basement and praying it doesn't hit your house and tear off the roof, waiting for the glass in the windows to shatter, because you are certain they will. This doesn't mean you do not have faith in your own children. It means you just know too much. Children make mistakes. It is not only about how hard you alone try. You have to have backup, you have to have other people watching.

Messy and complicated, that is how so many women label their lives as mothers, working outside the home or not, whether they are single or married, healthy or sick. I find that too simplistic and leaning negative.

I believe it mattered that I was able to forge a career from writing and teaching with the soul-deep belief in the sanctity of story. I write about my life not because I think I am so utterly fascinating, but because I think there are many women like me who have not had the platform to tell their stories and to share their truths. And in our true stories, we share connection. We glimpse hope.

Throughout our house are medals from wrestling tournaments on ribbons hanging in the kitchen, in each son's room, in drawers and cabinets, on bookshelves. Wrestling was a part of their lives at a critical time for each of them. I was not the most important person to them and for that, I am forever in debt. In our house there are trophies and wall plaques, framed brackets from tournaments, photos of hands raised in the air in victory. They earned them all.

I know I was lucky. I had my brothers and sisters who always helped me. My brother Paul helped me so often, I do not know what I would have done without his assistance. My sisters Madeleine and Maureen as well. But for my sons, I was their mother but also the outsider. It's not that I am so tied to gender roles; it's just that with raising three men, I needed a translator.

Coach Powell was that person. We still e-mail back and forth. He is semiretired, handing the title of head coach to Paul Collins.

But Powell will always be the heart and soul of the team. Powell sees Weldon often as Weldon lives back in Chicago and helps out as an assistant coach for wrestling at the high school. I see Powell at fundraisers with his wife and he always wants to know how the boys are doing. How the men are doing. He loves them, and I know that in my bones.

Powell has been in remission for the last year or so. He looks like himself, healthier and stronger, laughs more often, appears to have a lighter heart. Powell and his wife, Elizabeth, had their first child in 2015, a son they named after his father.

ACKNOWLEDGMENTS

P apa Bill died before any of my sons were born; my father would have assuredly adored them. My late mother, whom the grandchildren all called Mama Pat, made me feel I could do anything I intended. Every moment of my life I felt sincerely loved by them. I still do. My sisters Mary Pat, Maureen, and Madeleine are always there for me and for my sons. My brothers Bill and Paul, especially Paul, exemplify the strength of kindness. I do not know what I would do without U.P., the nickname my sons have for their beloved Uncle Paul. He helps me daily.

Caryn Ward sat with me in high school gyms for more than a decade as we screamed and cheered on each of our three sons from youth wrestling though high school. We worked together and carpooled on I-290 for many years solving the world's and our own problems on the commute. She is a fine editor and better friend. I am grateful to her for so many things, not least is her youngest son, Sam, who is Colin's best friend. Sue Schmidt and Lisa Lauren continually make me laugh. My college roommate Dana Halsted knows me as well as my sisters do. And I am grateful for her honesty and deep friendship.

Linda Berger, Diane Frisch, and Julie Shelgren have been offering their love and generous advice as we all have worked to raise our sons for the past two decades since we were Mets Moms in Oak Park youth T-ball.

Most Thursday evenings I am huddled with my writing group—Elizabeth Berg, Veronica Chapa, Arlene Malinowksi, Marja Mills, and Pamela Todd. For years in our group, Nancy Horan helped shaped me as a writer as well. Katherine Lanpher, Susy Schultz, Deborah Douglas, Alicia Shepard, and Teresa Puente are journalists I respect immensely and dear friends who offer honest feedback and laughter.

At the Medill School of Journalism at Northwestern University, Jack Doppelt, Karen Springen, Susan Mango Curtis, Michael Deas, and Craig Duff were forever supportive and encouraging. Dan Linzer, provost at Northwestern, and Lindsay Chase-Landsdale, associate provost, saw the value of my expertise and gave me the chance to work with the talented faculty through The OpEd Project's Public Voices Fellowship. I am grateful to Katie Orenstein, founder of The OpEd Project, for creating the opportunity for me to help others share their ideas with the world.

My doctors, Lauren Streicher, Kambiz Dowlat, and Joan Werber, are each exquisite examples of professional excellence and empathy; I owe them my life and my health and am grateful for who they are and what they have done for me.

Coach Mike Powell arrived in the lives of my sons as a man of integrity and intense personal courage. I am grateful for all he has done for my boys as well as for his candor and friendship. Hundreds of young men look to him for guidance, inspiration, and friendship, and his induction into the National Wrestling Hall of Fame in 2015 points to his enormous influence.

Lisa Reardon, my editor at Chicago Review Press, was wise and encouraging as she helped me clarify this complicated story. I am extraordinarily grateful.

My sons are true blessings; Weldon, Brendan, and Colin enrich my life and my heart beyond measure.